Praise for Planting the
An Integrative Approach to Fertility Care

"This book's eight chapters are a great resource that helps to answer questions I often hear in clinic like: 'When is the best time for us to have sex each month? What can Chinese medicine do for me? What do I do once I become pregnant?' The book clearly explains both the Traditional Chinese Medicine (TCM) and conventional medicine approaches, and how they can work well together. Once pregnant, the book then provides guidance on how TCM supports a healthy pregnancy. This is easy bedside reading with pragmatic solutions to help you feel empowered in your fertility journey."
– Lee Hullender Rubin, DAOM, LAc, FABORM, international lecturer, expert clinician, and published clinical researcher

"The synergy of Eastern and Western medicine to address fertility issues is expertly presented by Dr. Lora Shahine and Stephanie Gianarelli, both highly regarded experts in the fertility field."
– Lynn Jensen, author of Yoga and Fertility: A Journey to Health and Healing

"Wonderful resource for my fertility patients! I really enjoyed reading this book as I have many patients who are interested in integrating acupuncture into their fertility treatment. As a physician, I appreciate the research presented in this book, and it helps me answer the questions my patients have about how Eastern medicine can be used to optimize their preconception health. I loved the chapters discussing diet and supplements for fertility/egg/sperm health– this is a hot topic and an important subject I discuss at all of my new patient consultations. I am excited to tell my patients about this book as I know that it will be an invaluable resource during their journey to start or complete their family."
– Kathleen O'Leary, MD, lieutenant colonel, MC, United States Air Force, reproductive endocrinologist, and medical director of the Women's Health Clinic at Wright-Patterson Medical Center in Dayton, Ohio

"Science-based research, East meets West, and user-friendly! *Planting the Seeds of Pregnancy: An Integrative Guide to Fertility* has excellent, science-based research, blends the Eastern and Western perspectives on fertility, and is user-friendly. I find this book easy to dip into as a resource, as well as being read from cover to cover. I hope the authors will continue to update the book

as new findings about fertility are discovered. This is a must-have for those who are beginning to think about conceiving and for those who are already well on their journey."
– Fiona McLeod, fertility support group facilitator and contributor to Still a Mother: Journeys Through Perinatal Bereavement

"I really enjoyed how this book combined Eastern and Western medicine. I found the dietary and supplement recommendations throughout the book to be very informative and useful. This is a great book not only for those going through fertility treatment but for anyone preparing for a healthy pregnancy."
– Tamara Tobias, reproductive RN and author of Fertility Walk: A Fertility Nurse's Guide Along Your Journey

PLANTING THE SEEDS OF PREGNANCY

An Integrative Approach to Fertility Care

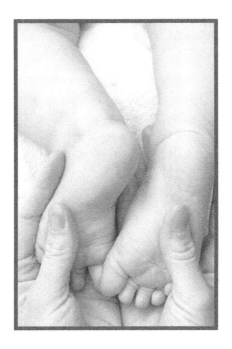

STEPHANIE GIANARELLI, LAC, FABORM
AND LORA SHAHINE, MD, FACOG

Seattle, Washington
2015

Planting the Seeds of Pregnancy: An Integrative Approach to Fertility Care
ISBN: 978-0-9963487-13

Contents

Forward: by Judy Kimelman, MD, FACOG 4

Preface: by Lora Shahine, MD, FACOG 5

Introduction: by Stephanie Gianarelli, LAc, FABORM 8

·♨·

Chapter One: Traditional Chinese Medicine: Overview and Use in Fertility Care 11

Chapter Two: Building Your Baby Bank Account with Traditional Chinese Medicine 17

Chapter Three: The Four Pillars of Fertility Enhancement 25

Chapter Four: Fertility Enhancing Supplements and the Science Behind Improving Egg Quality 36

Chapter Five: Optimizing Natural Conception 56

Chapter Six: Your First Acupuncture Treatment 65

Chapter Seven: Assisted Reproductive Technology: The Western Approach to Fertility Treatment 69

Chapter Eight: TCM Fertility Enhancement for ART 83

Chapter Nine: I'm Pregnant! Now What? 87

·♨·

Appendix One: What is Your Chinese Medicine Diagnosis? 96

Appendix Two: TCM Dietary Guidelines 104

Appendix Three: Understanding Your Digestion Through The Middle Burner 106

Appendix Four: The Issue of Pesticides and Chinese Herbal Medicine 108

Appendix Five: Finding Your Fertility Care Providers 110

·♨·

Glossary of Terms and Acronyms 113

Research, Sources and Additional Information 118

About The Authors 136

Index 140

Forward by Judy Kimelman, MD, FACOG

Traditionally, Western and Eastern medicine have been mutually exclusive of each other, but Stephanie and Lora present the reader with a world where the two can be integrated, with wonderful results.

In this book, the authors share scientific studies and anecdotes to support the philosophy of Traditional Chinese Medicine while explaining the benefits of Western medicine. For anyone in the throes of an infertility workup or treatment, they will find a different approach to a heavily medicalized field.

As a physician trained in Western medicine, it can be difficult to endorse a treatment for which there is no Western medical or strict scientific explanation. In the mid 80's during a medical school interview, I was asked how I thought acupuncture worked. It is a question I have pondered many times over the years. Now, as a practicing obstetrician for over 25 years, I have come to realize it does not matter exactly how it works, it matters that it does work. Stephanie and I have shared patients together for years and at times have had some miraculous results.

Western medicine approaches the issue of infertility by looking for a specific diagnosis and treatment while Eastern medicine brings a holistic approach, looking at nutrition, stresses, toxins and the impact of our environment. Blending the two together not only improves the end result but also helps women deal with the stress during an emotional process.

This book is a much-needed addition for those couples facing the challenges of trying to get pregnant and stay healthy in the process. It is wonderful to have a resource that explains both approaches and allows the patient to move easily between the two.

Dr. Judy Kimelman obtained her medical degree from Stanford Medical School. She is the current chair of the American College of OB/GYN Washington Section and a board member of the Washington State Medical Association and the Seattle GYN Society.

Preface by Lora Shahine, MD, FACOG

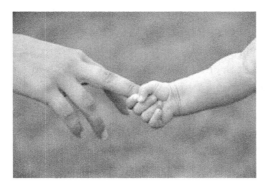

Western and Eastern medicine have two very different approaches to infertility, but that does not mean that these two methods have to be exclusive of each other. I am a physician trained in Western medicine and have never formally studied Traditional Chinese Medicine (TCM) and acupuncture, but I have shared patients with Eastern medicine providers and seen benefits like lower stress levels, regulation of menstrual cycles, and successful pregnancies.

The hesitation of Western medicine providers to embrace TCM is partially due to the historical lack of peer-reviewed evidence to support its success in patients, but this is starting to change.

My first exposure to Eastern medicine was one of the first attempts to study TCM with Western medicine techniques. In the summer of 1999, I did an internship in the oncology department at the University of California at San Francisco (UCSF), helping with a research study designed to examine the use of TCM in breast cancer.

The team at UCSF was using Western medical technology (blood tests, mammograms) to measure response to TCM treatments (herbs, acupuncture) in women with stage IV (end stage) breast cancer. The TCM provider was Yeshi Dhonden, a Buddhist monk and personal physician to the Dalai Lama from 1960-1980, who specializes in treating cancer with TCM techniques.

What I saw that summer was drastically different from anything I had ever seen in my medical training. Yeshi Dhonden would examine patients' tongues and pulses and prescribe herbs that smelled horrible. We did not cure breast cancer that summer – some patients had improvements in their disease (smaller masses on mammograms) and others progressed/worsened. We did, however, start a conversation (at least a segment on CBS's *60 Minutes*). I returned to medical school at the end of the internship energized by what I had seen, but faced less than enthusiastic scrutiny from my mentors and peers at the project presentation.

I returned to UCSF for my medical training for residency in Obstetrics and Gynecology and observed patients using moxibustion to turn babies from breech presentation to vertex presentation and acupuncture to induce labor. I completed my fellowship in Reproductive Endocrinology and Infertility at Stanford University and saw some patients using TCM and acupuncture in conjunction with intrauterine inseminations and IVF. My personal observation during this time was that the two practices tolerated each other but remained skeptical of each other.

I continued my casual observations of TCM and acupuncture when I moved to Seattle to practice. As a Western fertility provider, I do a standard evaluation of fertility and recommend Western techniques of ovarian stimulation, intrauterine inseminations, and IVF. One of the most common questions I hear after I give recommendations or when I am discussing a failed treatment plan from patients is, "What else can I do?"

A lot of my patients are very interested in methods for improving egg quality. It is widely understood that women are born with a finite number of eggs and that as they age, fewer of these eggs are able to result in a successful pregnancy. As we learn more about genetics and its role in fertilization, implantation, and healthy pregnancies, women are asking about methods that could potentially improve fertility by improving function at the level of DNA, mitochondria, and chromosomal function.

Patients ask about supplements, acupuncture, and alternative treatments every day. I tell them I have had patients benefit from TCM and acupuncture but that it may not be for everyone. Fertility treatment already involves multiple appointments and significant out of pocket costs—increasing time out of work for acupuncture treatments and the additional cost of alternative therapies can increase the already time-consuming and expensive fertility journey. I also explain that evidence showing the benefits of Eastern medicine alternatives is limited (although this is starting to change).

I first started working with Stephanie Gianarelli when she referred a patient to me for treatment. I appreciated her team approach to fertility care. She was the first TCM provider who had ever referred a patient to me directly and I appreciated her respect for Western medicine techniques. She and I agreed that Eastern and Western techniques do not have to be exclusive of each other and that each method can benefit patients in different ways. I appreciate Stephanie's focus on the evidence surrounding TCM and acupuncture. She is continuing the conversation started with the UCSF breast cancer project from 1999: Western research methods to examine Eastern medicine techniques.

Our collaboration on this book developed little by little over time. Stephanie had been working on a guide to the TCM approach to fertility for years and asked me to write a chapter on Western fertility treatment. After she asked me to look at other chapters and provide my perspective, we realized that the work had turned into a true collaboration. Through this guide we hope to continue the conversation between Eastern and Western Medicine approaches to fertility care. The book can be used as a guide for anyone considering fertility treatment either just starting out or those in treatment who want to explore options and enhance what they are already doing.

Enjoy!

Introduction by Stephanie Gianarelli, LAc

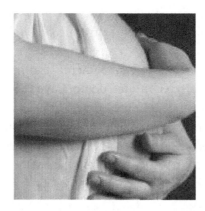

At 35 years old, Meghan came to my clinic trying to get pregnant. She and her husband had been actively trying for eight years, had been married for ten, and had never used birth control. She had stage three endometriosis, which had been removed twice, and a lime-sized fibroid removed the year prior. Her fertility lab work (a day 3 FSH of 14.8 and an AMH 0.3) was showing diminished ovarian reserve.

Meghan had been to two different fertility clinics. Both had told her she was not a good candidate for IVF and suggested that she use eggs from a donor instead of attempting IVF with her own. She admitted to having night sweats and insomnia, two possible symptoms of perimenopause. She had managed to get pregnant once, but that pregnancy had ended in miscarriage at seven weeks.

Meghan came to my clinic like many of my patients do—desperate to have a baby and feeling hopeless. We went through a thorough Chinese medicine diagnosis process and started her on acupuncture and Chinese herbal medicine. We added supplements, adjusted her nutrition, and suggested some lifestyle changes. She also began taking her basal body temperature every morning to give us more information. Within three months, she was pregnant. She went on to deliver a healthy baby girl.

I have to admit that I had forgotten Meghan's story until recently, when she returned to see me. It was six years later, and she was pregnant naturally without actively trying. With twins!

Although hers is a bit of a dramatic story, Traditional Chinese Medicine can result in major changes in people's fertility, and in many cases, the end result is a baby in their arms.

Maybe you are beginning to wonder if you need help getting pregnant, or maybe, like Meghan, you have been struggling through various fertility treatments for years without success. Maybe you are just beginning down the path to pregnancy, or perhaps you are trying for baby number two. No matter where you are on your family building journey, this book can help.

In contrast to Western medicine, which focuses on identifying and treating specific diagnoses, the ultimate goal of Traditional Chinese Medicine (TCM) is to optimize all aspects of body, mind, and spirit. Whether you are trying naturally or with Western fertility procedures, it is important that both parents strive for optimal health in order to increase the chances of conception, potentially increase the quality of both egg and sperm, help carry the pregnancy to term, and optimize the health of the future child.

Since many people choose to combine Eastern and Western fertility methods, Dr. Lora Shahine, board certified reproductive endocrinologist and expert on Western fertility care, has joined me in the writing of this book. Using the time-tested methods of TCM fertility enhancement, as well as modern advances in science, we've worked together to bring you the best that the East and West has to offer in a format that is easy to read and implement.

In this book, we will cover optimal nutrition, supplements, and lifestyle choices for increased fertility and enhanced sperm and egg quality, as well as overall health for both mother and father. We will discuss how to monitor your menstrual cycles for irregularities and time intercourse to improve natural conception. We will review how TCM helps enhance fertility and how it supports women throughout their pregnancy and after they give birth.

We will also walk you through what to expect at your first acupuncture appointment and help demystify the Western medical approach to fertility evaluation and treatment by reviewing which options are available in addition to or in conjunction with a TCM approach to fertility care.

Throughout the book, we offer tips and anecdotes from our personal practices, and in chapter nine, we've included insights into a Western medicine approach to prenatal care from Dr. Judy Kimelman, a practicing obstetrician and the current chair of the American College of OB/GYN Washington Section.

At the end of the book, we provide an extensive list of resources on the topics covered, including the most up-to-date research on egg and sperm quality and fertility enhancement. You'll also find appendices with information that will help you find a fertility care provider, figure out your TCM diagnosis, choose safe supplements, and eat to optimize health and fertility.

Let's get started!

1

Traditional Chinese Medicine: Overview and Use in Fertility Care

Traditional Chinese Medicine (TCM) is a comprehensive system of medical care that originated 2000-3000 years ago and has been evolving ever since. TCM uses acupuncture, Chinese herbal medicine, nutritional therapy, and lifestyle modifications to restore and maintain balance with a goal of bringing patients to a state of overall well being.

As a holistic form of medicine, TCM focuses on wellness rather than disease and can find and correct subtle imbalances in the body before they turn into illness. By treating patients into a state of optimal health, TCM helps improve the chances of conception by restoring balance in the body and mind, thus eliminating issues that may be leading to infertility.

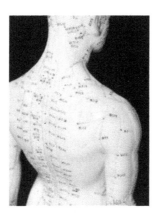

Finding a Fertility Acupuncturist

In China, some TCM practitioners specialize in certain areas of health, similar to medical doctors in the United States. Specialties in gynecology and treatment for infertility have a long history in Chinese medicine—the first obstetrics and gynecology herbal medicine book, *The Complete Book of Effective Prescriptions for Diseases of Women*, was written in 1237 AD. Through all of this time, this ancient medicine has offered powerful tools to help people achieve their dreams of having children.

You are probably more familiar with the term acupuncturist than TCM practitioner, and therefore we are going to use the term acupuncturist in this book when we are referring to a TCM practitioner. For the purpose of fertility enhancement with TCM, you want to find an acupuncturist who not only specializes in fertility care but also has the herbalist training necessary to be a full TCM provider. (See Appendix Five, "Finding Your Fertility Care Providers," for tips on choosing a good fertility acupuncturist and reproductive endocrinologist).

People go to fertility acupuncturists for a variety of reasons. Some want the non-invasive, holistic approach to their health that TCM provides, and others use TCM in conjunction with Western fertility treatments, such as intrauterine inseminations (IUIs), in vitro fertilization (IVF), or other assisted reproductive technologies. Some people seek TCM as a starting point for care and others find it after conventional treatments have failed. Wherever you are on your journey to parenthood, TCM can help.

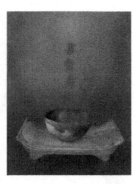

Research studies on the effects of TCM and fertility, pregnancy, and postpartum are encouraging. Studies have shown that all parameters of semen (including sperm count, motility, and morphology) can be favorably affected by TCM. Female fertility can be enhanced by TCM as well. There have been numerous studies on how TCM can regulate the cycles of women with polycystic ovary syndrome (PCOS) and boost success rates with assisted reproductive technologies such as IVF.

For a list of research on the benefits of TCM for fertility enhancement, pregnancy, and postpartum issues, see the resources section at the end of this book. The research is categorized by topic, and a synopsis of each study is given.

The Acupuncture Procedure

When you visit your fertility acupuncturist, they will look to the specific model of health that TCM measures everybody against and identify where you are out of balance. The focus of your treatment will be to correct any imbalances. Because it views the body and mind as inseparable, TCM is effective for addressing both physical and emotional imbalances, both of which can affect fertility.

Acupuncturists use the body's energetic framework to balance the flow of Qi (vital energy or life force, pronounced "chee") in the body. If the body's Qi is deficient, in excess, not moving, or scattered, disease often follows. By inserting thin, sterile, single-use needles into acupuncture points on Qi pathways (called meridians), the acupuncturist can help balance the flow of Qi, which in turn improves health. Because of its ability to detect subtle imbalances, Chinese medicine can help prevent illness before it progresses to the stage of disease.

Once you begin working with an acupuncturist, you can tell that you are progressing because you will start feeling better and have more energy. Your sex drive may increase, your sleep may improve, feelings of stress may decrease, your menstrual cycles and digestion may become more regular, and your symptoms of premenstrual syndrome (PMS) may disappear. As your symptoms decrease, you begin to move closer to that ideal model of health—and a step closer to conception.

A 43-year old woman came to me for help trying to conceive. She was solely focused on getting pregnant but was suffering from multiple symptoms, including low sex drive, fatigue, and severe edema. After we started working together, many of her symptoms began to disappear, her energy returned, her digestion improved, and her sex drive came back. She began to have fertile cervical fluid again, like she used to when she was in her twenties. She came to realize that getting her health back was a wonderful side benefit of fertility enhancement acupuncture. —Stephanie

When Should I See a Fertility Acupuncturist?

If you are trying to get pregnant or if you plan to start trying in the near future, it's best to get started with a fertility acupuncturist right away. The benefits of TCM treatment take time, so the sooner you start, the better. Ideally, you want to start seeing an acupuncturist at least three months before you start trying to conceive. Taking steps to improve your health is a great idea at any time, but if you think you may want to get pregnant in the future, even if that time is years away, it's best to begin focusing on your health now.

> **The top four reasons to see a fertility acupuncturist before trying to conceive:**
> 1. To increase the chances of conception.
> 2. For guidance on creating your roadmap to a healthy baby.
> 3. To get as healthy as possible for the ongoing health of your future children.
> 4. For emotional support along the way to becoming a parent.

What If I Have Fertility Issues?

These days, many patients choose to add acupuncture and herbs to other fertility treatments, with great results. Chinese medicine integrates very well with Western medical practices, and fertility acupuncturists are well versed in how to integrate Eastern and Western medicine safely and effectively.

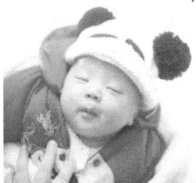

Whether you have been diagnosed with infertility or you want to enhance your fertility, the goal of TCM is always to help you become as healthy as possible in a holistic manner, which means that TCM is always a good choice.

As a reproductive endocrinologist, I provide a Western approach to fertility treatment, including diagnosing and treating causes of infertility and recurrent pregnancy loss. However, I have seen benefits to the holistic approach that TCM and Eastern medicine provide my patients. The two approaches do not have to be exclusive of each other, and I hope patients can find a balance between an East and West approach along their fertility journey. —Lora

TCM can often help with the following *female* diagnoses:
- ❏ Poor egg quality and diminished ovarian reserve (DOR)
- ❏ Recurrent pregnancy loss (RPL)
- ❏ Premature ovarian failure (POF)
- ❏ Polycystic ovary syndrome (PCOS)
- ❏ Luteal phase defect (LPD)
- ❏ Failed assisted reproductive technology (ART) or in vitro fertilization (IVF)
- ❏ Endometriosis
- ❏ Autoimmune issues
- ❏ Thin endometrium (uterine lining)
- ❏ Ovarian cysts
- ❏ Anovulation (no ovulation), irregular ovulation, and irregular menstrual cycles
- ❏ Tubal disease
- ❏ Unexplained infertility
- ❏ Feelings of anxiety, depression, or stress around infertility

A spunky pastor's wife came into my office one day for her first visit. She already had two children, but a subsequent surgery left her with blocked tubes. She and her husband very much wanted a third child. I explained her options to her: IVF, which bypasses the tubes altogether, or our natural approach to unblocking tubes. I've learned over the years to offer the natural approach, even though it is very labor intensive, because it often works. So I told her what it would entail—herbs taken internally, castor oil packs on the low abdomen, abdominal massage, and herbal enemas. "What did you just say? Herbal enemas? Where?" the pastor's wife asked, not all that sweetly. I explained it to her, thinking she would decline. She didn't. She did everything I asked her to do, and then, after two months of intense, at-home treatment, she did 20 hours of fertility-based physical therapy to unblock her tubes. Within three

TCM can often help with the following *male* diagnoses:
- ❑ Poor sperm parameters, due to less than optimal vasectomy reversal or varicocele (enlargement of the veins within the scrotum)
- ❑ Unexplained poor sperm parameters (sub-optimal semen analysis results)
- ❑ Autoimmune issues, such as anti-sperm antibodies
- ❑ Erectile dysfunction
- ❑ Incomplete liquefaction (seminal fluid should liquefy within one hour at room temperature)
- ❑ Prostatitis (inflammation of the prostate gland)
- ❑ Feelings of anxiety, depression, or stress around infertility

Scott was sent into my office by his wife. He had never been to an acupuncturist, but he had just found out that he had a low sperm count. Although he was a little skeptical, he was willing to try TCM. He had classic signs of Kidney Essence Deficiency, including low back pain, knee pain, excess nighttime urination, and some diminished hearing. I put Scott on a classic herbal formula focused on replenishing his Kidney Essence, and his sperm count doubled within three months. His wife was pregnant soon afterwards.
—Stephanie

In the next chapter, we will look at how the body prepares for and supports a pregnancy through the lens of Traditional Chinese Medicine.

2

Building Your Baby Bank Account with Traditional Chinese Medicine

We've discussed how the goal of TCM is to help both men and women be as healthy as possible—not only to aid in conception but to optimize the health of the future child. We've also covered how you can work with a fertility acupuncturist to increase your chances of conception. Now let's look at making a baby through the lens of Traditional Chinese Medicine.

The Organ Systems in TCM

Rooted in the philosophy of Taoism, TCM is based on the theory that the body's organ systems mutually support each other to achieve and maintain health and balance.

In TCM, the organ systems are a complex of structures and energy that work together and include both the actual organ as well as the corresponding meridian. Within the organ systems, the organs themselves, for the most part, do what they do in western medicine, but the organ systems as a whole have additional functions that take the whole person into account. (So when we talk about the Liver, for instance—as opposed to the liver—we're talking about the Liver Organ System).

When you go to see an acupuncturist, they will look for certain patterns of symptoms that speak to the presence of an imbalance in specific organ systems, measuring you against an ideal model of health. Health is achieved with a balance of these organ systems, and disease originates from an imbalance of these organ systems.

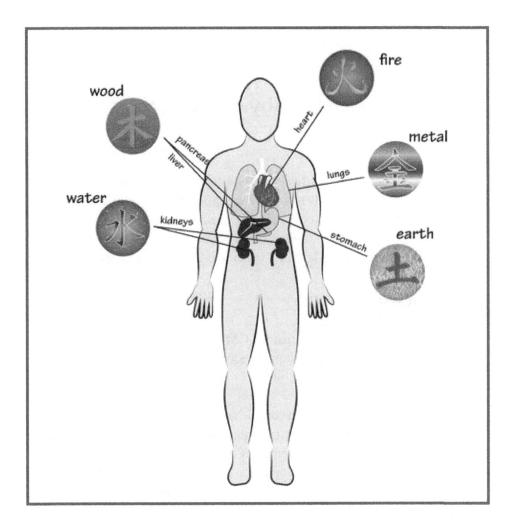

The organs communicate with each other through a vital energy called Qi, and a disruption in the flow of Qi (or communication between organ systems) will result in illness. TCM achieves balance through several treatment options, including acupuncture, herbs, and a holistic approach to health that includes diet, exercise, and lifestyle modifications.

Because Chinese medicine is holistic, all aspects of ourselves are reflected within its framework. Our personalities and emotions find a home within the different organ systems of the body. For example, when one worries a lot, has digestive upset with stress, and craves sugar, those symptoms signal an imbalance in the Spleen Organ System. The Liver Organ System is associated with detoxification, just as it is in Western medicine, but in TCM, it is responsible for emotional as well as physical toxins. (See Appendix One,

"What is Your Chinese Medicine Diagnosis," for an overview on these symptom groups and their corresponding diagnoses).

Since all of the major organ systems are important to maintaining your health and achieving a healthy pregnancy, the goal of the fertility acupuncturist is to balance the organ systems to improve all aspects of fertility to help a couple conceive. Let's take a look at each of the major organ systems in TCM and how they are involved in fertility.

The Liver

The Liver gets rid of toxins in the body. What that means in practical terms is that the Liver Organ System has to process all of our emotional as well as physical toxins. These could be toxins that we have ingested through eating or breathing, toxins absorbed through our skin, toxins that are endogenous waste products (like surging hormones), or toxins that are the result of strong emotions.

Even if we have never heard of the concept that some emotions can be toxic to the body, research shows that stress, grief, and joy can leave powerful physical footprints (Cohen et al. 2012), and long-standing stress has been shown to lower a woman's fertility outcomes (Louis et al. 2011).

In addition to detoxification, the Liver is also in charge of making sure that transitions occur in the body. For women, that includes ovulation and regular cycles. When a woman's body is getting ready for its monthly cycle, Liver energy is needed to make that happen. When PMS symptoms occur, this is a sign that the Liver is being overtaxed, usually from excess toxins, physical or energetic, bogging down the Liver's capacity to function. When this happens, the Liver doesn't have enough energy to get the cycle flowing smoothly, and PMS symptoms are often the result.

Irritability and anger are emotions of the Liver Organ System, and these emotions are another way for us to know that the Liver is being overtaxed. Other symptoms of a stagnant Liver are various types of headaches and stress-induced neck and shoulder tension. Acupuncture is great at moving Liver Qi and reducing Liver Qi stagnation symptoms like PMS.

The Heart

The Heart Organ System is important when it comes to fertility because the Heart lends its Blood to the uterus, and this allows conception to occur. (In TCM, Blood transports nourishment to the body and energy to the spirit).

In TCM, there is a meridian that directly connects the Heart to the reproductive complex (the uterus and the ovaries). Anxiety can negatively affect the Heart, revealing a direct correlation between our emotions and fertility. If anxiety is weakening the Heart energy, it is less able to nourish the reproductive organs. TCM practitioners are trained to look for and treat this potential emotional factor of infertility.

The Spleen

The Spleen Organ System is in charge of digestion. This organ system helps you get the most nutrients out of the food and drink you ingest. These nutrients are essential to life and get broken down into Qi and Blood in TCM. They are also necessary for conception to occur.

Worry damages the digestive tract. The digestion and especially the stomach are meant to remain warm in order to be able to break down food. For this reason, TCM advocates eating warm, cooked foods in order to help the digestive system break down foods into nutrients.

For more information about the digestive system, see Appendix Three, "Understanding Your Digestion Through The Middle Burner."

The Lungs

The Lungs are important in that they bring Qi (in the air we breathe) into our system and disperse it throughout our bodies. Although the Lungs are crucial for life and therefore fertility, they are often seen as less important in TCM than the other major organs in the treatment of infertility.

The Kidneys

In TCM, the Kidneys house our "Essence," which is thought of as the root of fertility for both men and women. It is sometimes helpful to think of your

Kidney Essence as your energetic "bank account." This bank account or Qi reserve is held in your Kidney Organ System. In TCM, your Essence is used to make sperm and eggs, and therefore, the health of your Kidney Essence dictates egg and sperm quality. Your Essence also houses your genetics, and just like your real bank account, it gets spent in your retirement or old age. Because of the importance of your Kidney Essence on your fertility, let's explore it in further depth.

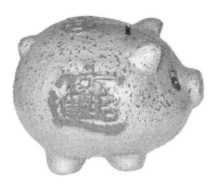

Your Baby Bank Account (Kidney Energy/Essence)

We all have a storehouse of Kidney Essence. The initial deposit into this account was made by our parents in the form of energy/Qi and genetics. After the initial gift of Essence from our parents (which can be large or small depending on our parents' genetics and their health at your conception), we are charged with the task of protecting that Essence by living a healthy lifestyle, as best we can.

When you live well and have a surplus of Qi at the end of the day, some of that Qi gets converted into Essence and is held in reserve in your Kidneys. It is from this bank account that babies are made. Both men and women use this energy to make a baby (as mentioned above, eggs and sperm come from Essence), but the woman has to further use her reserves in order to grow, deliver, and then potentially breastfeed the child.

When we speak of egg and sperm quality in Chinese medicine, we are speaking about the strength of our Kidney Essence. When you work to build your Kidney Essence, it is purported that you can improve egg and sperm quality—and some research is beginning to come out to corroborate this point of view.

In 2009, *Fertility and Sterility* published research that demonstrated biochemical changes in IVF patients treated with acupuncture, specifically the Cridennda Magarelli Acupuncture Protocol (CMAP). These changes were in the stress hormones prolactin and cortisol. This was the first paper to demonstrate a biochemical mechanism that may explain the beneficial effects of TCM in the form of acupuncture on IVF outcomes (Magarelli et al. 2009). Another study that came out in early 2015 seems to suggest that changes in cortisol levels (in the way that the CMAP protocol affected cortisol) may influence egg quality (Simerman et al. 2015). If you put these two studies together, you begin to see the power TCM has to affect change in the body, in this case, specifically egg quality.

TCM practitioners think about egg quality in terms of Kidney Energy or Essence. There are lifestyle choices that build Essence and some that deplete our reserves. Ideally, you want to build your reserves before trying to conceive, not only to enhance your fertility, but also to pass along the healthiest Qi that you can to your child.

From the Western side, it has been recently proven that the health of the parents at conception affects which genes get turned on and off in the child (Teh et al. 2014). This is called epigenetics, and it means that the health of both parents at conception directly affects the health of the child. This is a concept that has been in TCM for centuries, if not millennia.

What depletes my baby bank account?
- ❑ Using caffeine to spend more energy than you actually have in a day.
- ❑ Lack of sleep (leaving no chance for your body to rebuild).
- ❑ Serious illness.
- ❑ Extreme fear: the adrenals sit right on top of the kidneys and govern our fight or flight response, which is activated by fear).
- ❑ A genetic predisposition to Kidney deficiency (recognized by congenital diseases).

What builds my baby bank account?

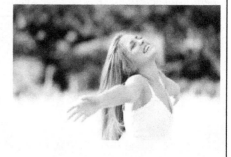

- ❑ Getting adequate rest, recognizing your limitations, and not over-scheduling your life.
- ❑ Rejuvenating exercises like yoga, Pilates, walking, hiking, etc. Now is not the time to start an intense, new exercise routine like training for a marathon or a new CrossFit class. Exercise relieves stress and can help maintain a healthy weight, but intense exercise that leaves you sore for days or severely fatigued is not healthy for anyone.
- ❑ Making healthy food choices, which can vary depending on your constitution.
- ❑ Eliminating toxins, such as tobacco, caffeine, and alcohol.
- ❑ Having a healthy relationship with stress. Well-meaning people often recommend 'taking a vacation' or 'just relaxing' to their family and friends who are struggling to conceive. This advice can often have the opposite effect, making us stress out about how stressed out we are. We cannot eliminate stress from our lives, but we can learn ways to cope with stress and decrease its impact on our health. Books, mind-body courses, group therapy, meditation, and counseling are some of the many resources that can help you find coping mechanisms for the daily stress we all encounter.

As you can see, living a healthy lifestyle and getting as healthy as possible before conception will help you keep reserves in your Kidney bank account, which will then help you when it comes to getting pregnant, and having more healthy Qi to share with your child.

TCM and acupuncture are relatively new concepts to me, especially in relationship to fertility and prenatal care. When Stephanie first started talking to me about Qi, kidney essence, and baby bank accounts, I was unsure–hesitant–because it sounded so different from my training in Western medicine. The more I listened, the more I understood that although Eastern medicine has a different approach and terminology, both Eastern and Western medicine have the same goal and message: helping people live a healthier lifestyle on the journey to parenthood. –Lora

3

The Four Pillars of Fertility Enhancement

Fertility enhancement relies on the time-tested four pillars of TCM treatment, as well as advances in other fields of complementary medicine. The term four pillars is used to explain several different concepts in TCM. For our usage, we are going to categorize the different interventions used by Traditional Chinese Medicine (TCM) to balance and strengthen the body.

The four pillars of Traditional Chinese Medicine include:
- ❏ Acupuncture
- ❏ Nutritional Recommendations
- ❏ Lifestyle Recommendations
- ❏ Chinese Herbal Medicine

The Four Pillars of Treatment

Working through the four pillars of treatment with a fertility acupuncturist is ideal because along with acupuncture, they can provide specific nutrition, herb and supplement recommendations for your personal situation. Supplements are not traditionally TCM but they incorporate modern medical research and will be covered in detail in the next chapter. In this chapter, we'll cover the universal guidelines you can start incorporating into your life that can help you start improving your fertility potential now!

Fertility acupuncturists recommend using the four pillars of treatment to strengthen fertility potential and balance overall health for at least three months before trying to conceive. Indeed, some fertility acupuncturists consider three months the absolute minimum preparation time needed and call this period pre-pregnancy treatment, as opposed to pre-conception planning, which can begin as early as two years prior to attempting to conceive.

While this timeline may not be realistic for everyone, you will benefit from balancing your health whenever you start. One study published in the medical journal *Fertility and Sterility* showed that only five weeks of acupuncture improved men's sperm counts and motility (Pei et al. 2005). TCM provides benefits from the moment you begin, and the sooner you begin, the better.

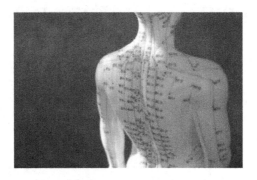

First Pillar of Treatment: Acupuncture

The first pillar of TCM treatment is acupuncture. This pillar also includes moxibustion (burning specific herbs at acupuncture points), among other modalities. As we discussed in Chapter One, acupuncture involves using hair-thin needles inserted at key points along the Qi pathways to encourage energy and blood flow throughout the body, including both the male and the female reproductive systems (although needles aren't put there!).

As a fertility treatment, acupuncture can help regulate ovulation, nourish the uterine lining, boost sperm parameters, and harmonize the endocrine system. (We will discuss what to expect at your first acupuncture appointment in Chapter Six).

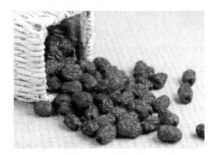

Second Pillar of Treatment: Nutritional Recommendations

One of the easiest ways to enhance your fertility and incorporate Chinese medicine into your life is through the foods you eat. In this section, we'll review the changes you can make to your diet to help increase your fertility. For more information, see Appendix Two, "TCM Dietary Guidelines." In addition to the guidelines listed below, your acupuncturist will make specific and effective recommendations based on your individual diagnosis.

> *A male patient came to us with a history of azoospermia, a condition in which there is no measurable level of sperm in semen. I say "history" because prior to seeing us, he changed his diet by cutting out sugar and processed foods and increasing his vegetable intake. He also started taking vitamins and fish oil. Within three months, the doctors found that he had sperm in his ejaculate! He had sperm where there was none, and the only change he had made at that point was improving his diet and taking supplements. He went on to further improve his sperm count. —Stephanie*

Nutrition for fertility for women and men

The following dietary guidelines will help improve your health no matter where you're at in life, but they are especially recommended if you are trying to conceive:

- ❏ **Eat organic, unprocessed foods**, including small amounts of hormone-free, organic meats.
- ❏ **Eat good monounsaturated fats** like (unheated) olive oil and avocados as they decrease inflammation in the body.
- ❏ **Eat good saturated fats** like butter (especially from grass-fed cows) and coconut oil. These fats provide the building blocks of hormones, constitute a large percentage of cell membranes, enhance the immune system, and provide fat-soluble vitamins, like vitamin A, D, E and K.
- ❏ **Keep your blood sugar stable**. When your blood sugar spikes, extra insulin is released, and if this continues, your body will start to ignore the extra insulin and you begin to become insulin resistant. This can eventually lead to type 2 diabetes.

Tips for keeping your blood sugar stable:
- ❑ Eat whole foods and avoid processed foods. Processed foods, such as white flour products, are very easy for the body to break down and can cause spikes in your blood sugar. Whole foods are harder to break down, which allows your body to absorb the glucose more slowly.
- ❑ Eat every 3 – 4 hours and don't skip breakfast.
- ❑ Eat moderate amounts of protein with each meal as they don't cause a rise in insulin levels.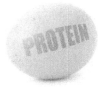
- ❑ Eat full fats as they also don't cause your insulin levels to elevate.

- ❑ **Drink bone broth**. Marrow is the only food we can consume that is actually Kidney Essence (remember your baby bank account). You can often find pre-made bone broth at a farmer's market or health food store. You can also make your own. Make sure to get organic, natural marrow bones. Drink half a cup 3 – 5 times a week.

Make your own bone broth. You can use this recipe as a base for any of your favorite broth-based soups, including pho!
Ingredients: 2 – 3 lbs marrow bones. (Opt for natural, organic marrow bones that come from local livestock that have been grass fed and grass finished).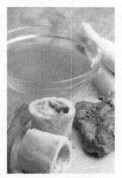
Directions: Crack the bones and put into a crock pot, cover with water and slow cook overnight. The next day, cool the soup and strain through cheesecloth. Let the broth cool to room temperature before placing it in the refrigerator. After it has cooled, skim off the fat and discard. Now the broth is ready to use in your favorite soup recipe. Extra broth may be placed in the freezer for future use.

- ❑ **Reduce alcohol consumption**. Research shows that there is an inverse relationship between alcohol consumption and embryo quality; more alcohol consumption by the woman leads to poorer embryo quality (Wdowiak et al. 2014).

❏ **Reduce coffee intake**. Although research on coffee in many different areas of health has been positive recently, most of the research doesn't support excess caffeine for fertility. Coffee contains alkaloids that are harmful to the system as they can damage cell membranes. Caffeine has also been linked to a decrease in the success rates of Assisted Reproductive Technologies (Klonoff-Cohen et al. 2002). In addition, a study has shown that drinking more than two cups of coffee per day during pregnancy (approximately 200 mg) may increase miscarriage rates (Weng et al. 2008). Caffeine intake during pregnancy can also have a negative effect on fetal growth (Momoi et al. 2008). From a TCM perspective, coffee negatively affects your Kidney Essence by expending energy that should be saved in your bank account. Think about caffeine as allowing you to spend more energy than you have in a given day—energy that comes from your Kidney Essence.

Reducing caffeine. If you choose to drink decaffeinated coffee, remember that it still contains harmful alkaloids. The caffeine content is greatly reduced, though, at only 2 mg of caffeine per cup, compared to an average of 50 – 95 mg in espresso and up to 200 mg in brewed coffee.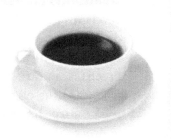
Make sure to stick to water process decaffeinated coffee. In standard decaf, the caffeine is removed using a toxic solvent called ethyl acetate, also found in nail polisher remover, which could also then be found in your coffee! Some people believe that the roasting burns off the chemicals, but it is best to avoid it altogether if you can.
Green tea is a good option if you feel the need for some caffeine. Although green tea does contain some caffeine (around 30 – 45 mg a cup), it also contains beneficial antioxidants and does not contain the harmful alkaloids found in coffee.

❏ **Eat foods high in antioxidants**. Anything dark and naturally colorful, especially beans and berries, is great for you. Antioxidants have demonstrated anti-inflammatory and anti-spastic effects and have been shown to be especially useful for fertility, as we will see in the next chapter.

❑ **Eat foods that decrease inflammation**, including those high in Omega-3 essential fatty acids. Many factors influence the inflammatory process in your body—stress, lack of exercise, genetic predisposition, and very importantly, nutrition. Just by adding the following foods and decreasing the amount of refined flours and sugars in your diet, you can begin to reduce inflammation throughout your body and thereby enhance your fertility.

Anti-inflammatory foods:

❑ **Eat foods containing Omega-3s** like cold-water oily fish (herring, mackerel, salmon, anchovies and sardines), grass-fed beef, walnuts, flax seeds, and pumpkin seeds.

❑ **Additional anti-inflammatory foods include**: olive and coconut oil, dark green veggies, cherries, blueberries, turmeric, ginger, garlic, green tea, and cruciferous veggies (such as broccoli, cauliflower, kale, and Brussels sprouts).

❑ **Make sure that you cook your cruciferous vegetables** (such as broccoli, cauliflower, cabbage, Brussels sprouts) if you have any type of thyroid issue. Uncooked cruciferous vegetables contain goitrogens that suppress thyroid function.

❑ **Avoid trans-fatty acids**, like those found in shortening, margarine, and hydrogenated vegetable oil as they impair the proper functioning of the immune and reproductive systems.

❑ **Drink enough water**. That amount varies from person to person. Research is showing that how much water people need to drink in order to stay hydrated depends on many variables, including constitution, activity level, and climate (American Society of Nephrology 2008).

❑ **Eat nuts and seeds** for the essential fatty acids, protein and zinc.

❑ **Take a multivitamin**. Supplement your diet (which should still be full of healthy, nutritious foods) with a natural, high potency multivitamin or prenatal vitamin and mineral complex with iron, folate, and B vitamins. Avoid 'one-a-day' vitamins as they are often of poor quality and are not readily absorbed. If you are taking one-a-day vitamins, break them in half and take half in the morning and the other half in the evening. When you run out, opt for vitamins that are in encapsulated powder form to increase your body's ability to absorb them. *Note*: supplements will be covered in more detail in the next chapter.

❏ **Take Fish Oil**. Fish oil improves blood flow to the ovaries and uterus (Lazzarin et al. 2009), boosts immune function (Gurzell et al. 2013), reduces inflammation, and helps your baby's neural development once you become pregnant (McNamara and Carlson 2006). Fish oil also contains omega-3 fatty acids, which work to improve sperm integrity (Safarinejad et al. 2010). If you are trying to get pregnant, many providers will recommend a daily dosage of 900 mg EPA, which helps reduce inflammation, and 600 mg DHA, which is needed for brain health in the pre-conception phase. *Note:* Vegetarian options include flax (flax contains ALA, which converts to EPA and DHA in small quantities) and algae (which provides mostly DHA). Consult with your healthcare provider before taking fish oil if you are taking blood thinners.

What to look for in a fish oil:
❏ **Fish oil made with smaller fish**, such as herring or anchovies, is better than oil from bigger fish because fish that are lower on the food chain contain less mercury. *Note:* getting enough selenium in your diet can help to reduce your body's absorption of mercury.
❏ **Make sure your fish oil is third-party tested**, has a Certificate of Analysis proving how clean it is, and that standards have been set by the IFOS (International Fish Oil Standards).
❏ **Make sure your fish oil is fresh** and not oxidized or it will cause inflammation instead of reduce it.

❏ **Avoid BPAs and phthalates**. Both Bisphenol A (BPA) and phthalates are colorless carbon compounds used in plastics that have been associated with miscarriage and lowered fertility rates (we'll discuss in more detail in the next chapter).

> *I fully support and encourage my fertility patients to eat the best they can by avoiding processed foods and choosing fresh, organic products if possible. Some recommendations, like avoiding smoking, are obvious to patients, but I get push back from patients on other suggestions like no alcohol or coffee (especially coffee, since my practice is in Seattle!). I advise patients to do the best they can and cut back on excessive intake of toxins. In my own practice, I have found that the patients who are resistant at first often feel so much better after changing some of their lifestyle choices that they make even more changes for the better. —Lora*

Third Pillar of Treatment: Lifestyle Recommendations

Making positive changes to your daily habits can enhance your fertility. For example, your fertility acupuncturist may suggest ways to reduce stress (or at least view it more positively), get more sleep, or get the right kind of exercise. If you are trying to get pregnant, the basic lifestyle recommendations in this section should help.

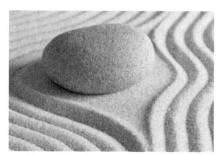

The lifestyle basics for women and men

❏ **Manage stress**. Think about stress as your body's way of preparing you to meet challenge. Stress can be impossible to avoid, and infertility is inherently stressful. However, research has been coming out that shows that our body's response to stress is not always a bad thing. The destructive part of stress seems to be how we think about it. When we perceive stress as destructive to the body, we increase our risk of disease, especially coronary heart disease (Richardson et al.

2012; Nabi et al. 2013). When we consider stress to be our body's way of preparing us to meet a challenge, stress seems to present less of a health risk (Keller et al. 2012). Therefore, working on how we think about stress is turning out to be more important than trying to avoid sometimes unavoidable stresses.

- ❏ **Be kind to yourself**. Try to get enough sleep, try not to work too much, and try to avoid anything too taxing to the immune system. In other words, give your body every chance to be at its strongest and healthiest so that it can nourish a child.

- ❏ **Unplug**. Disconnect from work, email, social media, and other obligations a little every day. We may feel like we are working hard when we are working many hours straight, but most people find that they can be more productive in a shorter amount of time when they plan for breaks/rest/time off from work.

- ❏ **Get your teeth cleaned**. The bacteria in your mouth can lead to periodontitis, which is inflammation of the tissue around the teeth. The bacteria can then spread to the rest of the body, increase inflammation and activate the immune system. Studies have shown that bad oral hygiene can increase the amount of time it takes to conceive (Nwhator et al. 2014).

- ❏ **Eliminate nicotine**. Research shows that cigarette smoking is linked to some decreased fertility in women (Håkonsen et al. 2014) and decreased sperm parameters (Al-Turki 2015; Kulikauskas et al. 1985).

Additional lifestyle suggestions for women

- ❏ **Enjoy low impact exercise**. Avoid sweating profusely, jarring or abdominal compression exercises, and high-impact activities such as running, particularly after ovulation, IVF transfer, or intrauterine insemination (IUI). Low impact activities such as yoga, swimming, walking, and the elliptical trainer are all good exercises for fertility.

My patients often ask me how much exercise is too much. I have seen too many patients completely give up exercise because they are worried they will do something to decrease chances of success only to become miserable without their usual exercise routine. High impact exercise with high bursts of energy (CrossFit) or excessively long workout routines (running 10+ miles) may alter hormonal levels and may impact

---

ovulation or progesterone production after ovulation, but most patients are not exercising enough to truly alter these hormones. Exercise is an excellent stress release, and I encourage low impact exercise. I find myself saying to patients trying to conceive, "this is not the time to start training for a marathon or start a new CrossFit/boot camp class," and I review their routine. If it sounds like high impact exercise too often, we'll discuss alternatives. —Lora

Additional lifestyle suggestions for men

❏ **Be careful with technology**. Do not rest laptops against the body or keep cell phones or other electronic devices in your pocket or on your belt loop. A study published in the *Journal of Andrology* in 2012 demonstrated a decrease in total sperm parameters (count, motility, and morphology) in relationship to sperm exposure to the radio frequency electromagnetic radiation emitted by cell phones, as well as to the duration of daily cell phone usage (La Vignera et al. 2012).

❏ **Talk to your doctor regarding any medications that may affect sperm count**. Some medications that can affect male fertility are prescribed for hypertension, peptic ulcers, ulcerative colitis, epilepsy, urinary function, gout, chemotherapy, anti-fungal medications, testosterone medications, and anabolic steroids.

❏ **Watch for and try to avoid other temporary causes of low sperm count**. Infections, increased stress, lack of sleep, and use of alcohol, tobacco, or marijuana can all decrease your sperm count. Be careful of exposure to radiation and to solvents, pesticides, and other toxins as well.

❏ **Reduce the amount of toxins you ingest**. Sperm are extremely sensitive to the effects of chemicals—in the environment and in food. We'll discuss the effects of toxins on sperm and egg quality in the next chapter.

Fourth Pillar of Treatment: Chinese Herbal Medicine

When appropriate, your acupuncturist will recommend customized herbal medicine treatment in the form of dried raw herbs, granules, tinctures, or pills as the fourth pillar of TCM treatment. Chinese herbal medicine is a very powerful way to make the body stronger and replenish what has been lost due to the pressures of modern life, disease, or poor lifestyle choices.

Chinese herbal medicine is a very important pillar of TCM for fertility enhancement. It has been the main treatment modality within TCM for fertility enhancement and has been used effectively to treat infertility for thousands of years. In the western world, TCM has focused more on acupuncture for infertile patients, although this has not been the case historically.

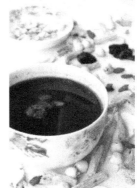

However, there is a body of research that shows how Chinese herbal medicine can enhance fertility. In one study (Ried and Stewart 2011), Chinese herbal medicine improved pregnancy rates two-fold in a four-month period. In the research section of this book, you'll find a whole section on Chinese herbal medicine and fertility for both men and women.

> *At our clinic, we use Chinese herbal medicine regularly for couples trying to conceive naturally. When couples are using Western fertility treatments, we use Chinese herbs leading up to ART and then discontinue their use during ART. An exception is made when the couple has several failed ART cycles. At that point, we will contact the fertility doctor (reproductive endocrinologist) to request that Chinese herbs be used in conjunction with ART. —Stephanie*

If you are thinking of getting pregnant, start today on these four pillars of treatment and you will be on your way to optimal fertility health!

4

Fertility Enhancing Supplements and the Science Behind Improving Egg Quality

In vitro fertilization (IVF) and other forms of assisted reproductive technology have revolutionized options for family building since the first IVF baby was born in 1978. While the advances in this technology over the last 40 years are incredible, there is one challenging issue that technology has not yet conquered, and that is diminished ovarian reserve.

Ovarian reserve is a term without a widely accepted, clear definition, but in general, women with good ovarian reserve have normal ovarian reserve testing, respond well to fertility treatments, and have a higher chance of conceiving naturally or with fertility treatments. Women with diminished ovarian reserve (DOR) usually have poor ovarian reserve testing, do not respond well to fertility treatment, and have a lower chance of conceiving naturally or with fertility treatment.

IVF can overcome blocked fallopian tubes, scarring from endometriosis, male factor infertility, and many other fertility challenges, but women with DOR are often told they are not good candidates for IVF and that they should consider other family building options, like IVF with donor eggs.

Current understanding of ovarian reserve is that in natural cycles, women have a pool of recruitable eggs and produce enough gonadotropin hormones to mature one of these eggs, which then hopefully ovulates. The eggs that reached the recruitable stage but were not selected that cycle are lost along with hundreds, maybe thousands, of premature eggs in the cycle. The next menstrual cycle, the whole process starts over with a different set of eggs.

In IVF, gonadotropin hormones are given at a higher dose than what the body can make in a natural cycle to help recruit and mature more than one egg in the pool of available eggs. The higher your ovarian reserve, the more eggs there are to be recruited, which increases the chance of more viable eggs that in turn increases your chance of success with IVF.

IVF does not change egg quality or quantity—it is a process that recruits the eggs that are available. If a patient has diminished ovarian reserve, they will have a poor response to gonadotropins, fewer eggs recruited, and a lower chance of success with IVF.

Egg Quality

As technology has advanced with IVF, we have learned more about fertility. As eggs age, fewer of them can do the genetic work possible to result in a successful pregnancy. This is why older women take longer to conceive, have a higher chance of miscarriage, and have a higher chance of having a child with Down's syndrome (although that risk is overall very small). To understand why this happens, we must review what happens with genetics at fertilization.

In every cell in our body, we have 23 pairs of chromosomes—one chromosome in each pair comes from the egg that made us and the other comes from the sperm. During fetal development, eggs within the female fetus develop up to a certain point in the womb and are then frozen in a genetic state (called meiosis) until later in life. Once the female starts ovulating, the ovulated egg has a lot of genetic work to do to get rid of half of its genetic content (its copies of chromosomes) in order to be ready to be fertilized by a sperm (which provides the matching second half of chromosomes).

If the egg makes any mistakes at ovulation (it holds on to an extra chromosome or gets rid of two copies of a chromosome), the resulting embryo will have an uneven number of chromosomes. Most embryos with an uneven number of chromosomes will not result in a viable pregnancy because the embryo will stop developing at some point, leading to a negative pregnancy test or miscarriage. Miscarriage is a common issue among women of all ages—15-25% of all pregnancies in women of all ages will end in miscarriage—but at 40 years old, the risk increases, and approximately 50% of positive pregnancy tests will not result in a live birth (ASRM 2012).

> *Once I teach my patients how complex genetics are to reproduction, they usually feel a sense of relief. At least there is a reason why some couples are struggling to complete their family. Not every egg or sperm is perfect, and as we age, fewer eggs and sperm are able to do the chromosome jigsaw puzzle needed to match up chromosomes. This knowledge helps many women with multiple miscarriages as well. —Lora*

A full 60-80% of first trimester miscarriages are due to an imbalance of chromosomes (Marquard 2010), but one chromosomal issue that can result in a live birth is Down's syndrome, which is caused by the embryo having three copies of the number 21 chromosome (trisomy 21). While the sperm can occasionally cause issues with chromosome number, chromosome mistakes are usually due to an error with the egg's genetic steps towards fertilization.

> For further reading, we recommend the book, *It Starts with the Egg* by Rebecca Fett. Rebecca is a former molecular biologist who struggled with her own diagnosis of diminished ovarian reserve and set out to review the literature and scientific evidence surrounding ways to improve egg quality. We have summarized the current knowledge regarding this topic here, but we refer you to Rebecca Fett's book for a more detailed discussion.

Supplements for Egg Quality

Many women who come into fertility clinics want to know if there is any way they can change their ovarian reserve. For instance, are there supplements or lifestyle changes that can alter the number or quality of available eggs? The answer is we do not know for sure, but there is research that suggests ways to possibly improve ovarian reserve.

> *In our clinic, we make use of the cutting edge research with fertility enhancing supplements while relying heavily on the millennia old Chinese medicine.*
> *—Stephanie*

In chapter three, we covered the basic lifestyle and diet suggestions for increasing fertility and improving egg quality. In this section, we will cover the supplements to take and the toxins to avoid to enhance your egg quality and increase your fertility. (Please note that vitamins and supplements should not replace good nutrition. Each person's supplemental needs are different and any recommendations or doses listed here are general guidelines—not medical advice. Please review any new supplements with your healthcare provider).

Although the current research around supplements and lifestyle changes as methods for improving fertility is encouraging, this is a relatively new area for

Western medicine. In order for a new treatment to be generally accepted and recommended to patients in Western medicine, usually there need to be several studies with large numbers of patients in different clinical settings that all agree that the intervention results in a significant benefit without significant risk to patients. FDA approval for a new medication, for example, can take years and substantial resources to be approved. Supplements do not fall under FDA regulation and do not require scrutiny before being sold and marketed to patients. This is important to understand when choosing a supplement since what is written on the label of a supplement bottle may not actually be what is in the supplement itself.

> *Personally, I am intrigued with the current evidence but I am cautious before recommending any new treatment. There are many examples in Western medicine of providers adopting a promising new drug or treatment for patients which later is found to be ineffective or even harmful. Fertility patients are particularly vulnerable—anxious to try anything that may help. I appreciate their position, but fads in fertility treatment come and go and I am surprised at the general assumption that a supplement or herb (anything over the counter) cannot be harmful. Supplements are not regulated and lack oversight and there are instances that when tested, supplements had little or none of the the advertised ingredients and instead contained potentially harmful fillers. I am following the evidence, willing to learn, and excited about the possibility that patients could do something to improve fertility beyond Western medical techniques, but I am cautious before adopting any new treatment for my patients.—Lora*

It's best to review supplement options with your fertility provider before taking them. Every patient and every situation is different and your provider should be able to help you decide on what is right for you.

Tips for choosing vitamins and supplements
❑ Be careful when choosing a vitamin. Supplements are not regulated by the FDA like medications are, and not all vitamins and supplements are equal. Some are inconsistent with ingredients or contain fillers that do not provide nutrition and in

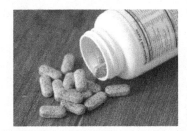

rare cases can be harmful if taken in excess.
- ❑ Do your own research or trust a professional.
- ❑ As a basic rule, avoid very inexpensive or generic brands.
- ❑ Read the labels to check for unnecessary ingredients and to make sure that the dosing of the various vitamins and minerals is high enough.
- ❑ Choose a multivitamin that needs to be taken multiple times a day. Our gut can absorb only small amounts of nutrition and vitamins at a time (especially vitamins C and B) so taking smaller doses multiple times throughout the day is a way to optimize intake.

Folate and Folic Acid

Folate and folic acid are forms of a water-soluble B vitamin. Folate occurs naturally in food, and folic acid (as the name is used in the supplement form) is the synthetic form of this vitamin. Besides being important for the health of the future child, folate is essential for DNA synthesis, which is key to egg quality and development. One study showed women taking additional folic acid supplements in IVF had better quality oocytes and more mature eggs (Szymanski and Kazdepka-Zieminska 2003). Mouse studies have shown that folate is essential for early embryo development due its role in DNA synthesis and repair (O'Neill 1998).

One study in humans showed that women had a lower incidence of children with Down's syndrome if they took supplemental folic acid (Blencowe 2010). Since Down's syndrome is a chromosomal mismatch, which usually occurs at the level of the egg at ovulation, Rebecca Fett in *It Starts with the Egg*, suggests there may be a link between adequate folic acid supplements and correct chromosomal processing within the egg (Fett 2014). There is certainly biologic plausibility of the role of folic acid in DNA replication and repair; however, more evidence is needed before we can make this assumption. For now, it is widely recommended that women who are trying to conceive take folate to prevent neural tube defects. If it helps with egg quality too, that would be a wonderful bonus.

Folic acid has been added to our foods by government mandate since 1998 to help reduce birth defects. There is now some concern that excess (synthetic) folic acid in the

> *bloodstream could be harmful (Deghan Manshadi et al. 2014), although the scientific debate on this is still going on (Vollset et al. 2013). Also, as we will discuss below, some patients may not be able to absorb folic acid due to the gene mutation MTHFR. For these reasons, at our clinic, we always recommend women take methylated folate (at 1000 mcg a day) rather than folic acid. —Stephanie*

Folate and MTHFR

When folic acid is taken as a supplement, it must be converted into the biologically active form 5-methyl tetrahydrofolate by the enzyme methylenetetrahydrofolate reductase, or MTHFR, in order to exert its functions. Essentially, MTHFR needs to add a methyl group or alter folic acid before it can be used in the body for DNA replication and other processes. The MTHFR enzyme is coded by the MTHFR gene, and up to 40% of the general population can have a mutation in this gene (Ueland et al. 2001). The defect in this gene results in a reduced function of the MTHFR enzyme, which means that up to 40% of the population will not process folic acid supplements adequately.

Women with one defect (heterozygous) in the MTHFR gene will be able to utilize only 65% of the folic acid supplement they take in regular prenatal vitamins and women with two defects (homozygous) will be able to utilize only 35% compared to women with no genetic defects in their MTHFR genes (Frosst et al. 1995; Van der Put et al. 1995). This discovery has led to the creation of methylated folic acid supplements in which the methyl group is already added. In theory, this methylated folic acid supplement should be easier to use and process in people with a defect in their MTHFR gene.

> ❏ **Food Sources of Folate**: To naturally increase your folate levels, eat unprocessed, organic foods with high levels of folate such as meat (liver, kidney, egg yolk), legumes (beans, lentils, peas), fruits (oranges, peaches, bananas) and vegetables (spinach, broccoli, cabbage, Brussels sprouts).
> ❏ **Tips for Folate Supplementation**: Recommended doses differ between studies and official guidelines, so you should review your needs with your fertility provider. In general, many providers recommend approximately 800-1000 mcg of methylated folate

(rather than folic acid) daily when trying to conceive and throughout pregnancy.

❑ **Potential Side Effects**: Potential side effects of taking too much folic acid include diarrhea, stomach cramps, nausea and/or irritability. Potential side effects from taking methylated folate include irritability, insomnia, muscle aches, headaches and/or anxiety.

Vitamin D

Vitamin D is a fat-soluble vitamin that is found in some food and supplements but is usually produced in our bodies when UV rays from sunlight trigger vitamin D synthesis from cholesterol in our skin. It is essential for helping with calcium absorption and maintaining bone health but also has important roles in our overall health. Vitamin D deficiency has been associated with increased risk for diabetes, cardiovascular disease, and cancer (Giammanco et al. 2015; Galesanu and Mocanu 2015), and adequate vitamin D replacement has been associated with improved mood (seasonal affective disorder/winter blues) and improved immune system function (Galesanu and Mocanu 2015).

In the female body, the active form of vitamin D is needed for everything from maturing eggs, preparing the uterus, assisting with embryo implantation, boosting the immune system to fight infections during pregnancy, and assisting in a healthy pregnancy.

Some studies suggest that vitamin D deficiency may be associated with decreased fertility and lower success with fertility treatments. Studies have also shown a higher rate of natural conception with higher levels of vitamin D (Ozkan et al. 2010). Other studies have shown higher fertilization rates, implantation rates, and pregnancy success rates with IVF in patients with adequate vitamin D levels (Rudick et al. 2012; Firouzabadi et al. 2014; Ozkan et al. 2010; Paffoni et al. 2014). Theories regarding the role of vitamin D in reproduction include its potential role in hormone production, uterine lining receptivity (Rudick et al. 2012), and egg development (Luk et al. 2012). Other studies have shown a direct relationship between vitamin D and anti-Müllerian hormone (AMH) production (Merhi et al. 2012).

Anti-Müllerian hormone (AMH) is produced by granulosa cells in the ovaries—the supporting cells of developing eggs. AMH levels decline with age and can be a sign of diminished ovarian reserve. Higher vitamin D levels have been associated with higher AMH levels (Merhi et al. 2012). Vitamin D has also been shown to improve male factor infertility, especially motility (Blomberg Jensen 2014).

Most people do not know they need vitamin D replacement since symptoms of vitamin D deficiency such as muscle weakness and pain only occur when levels are severely low. A blood test for vitamin D levels (called serum 25 Hydroxyvitamin D) is the most accurate way to know whether you are vitamin D deficient. A level of less than 30 ng/mL is generally considered too low.

Adequate sun exposure for vitamin D synthesis differs by a person's age, skin color, and overall health. In general, 30 minutes of sun exposure twice a week without sunscreen may be enough for some people, but too much UV exposure is associated with skin cancer. Many health professionals recommend vitamin D supplements, especially in the winter months.

❏ **Food Sources of Vitamin D**: Vitamin D can be found in some foods like fish, egg yolks, and vitamin D fortified dairy products.
❏ **Tips for Vitamin D Supplementation**: Find a supplement formulated in oil and eat with a fat-containing meal (fat helps with better Vitamin D absorption). A starting dose is usually around 3000 mg per day (check with your healthcare provider for specific dosages).
❏ **Potential Side Effects**: Too much vitamin D can result in excessive levels of calcium and symptoms of gastrointestinal and kidney problems, so before you start taking high doses, check with your healthcare provider.

Coenzyme Q10 (CoQ10)

This enzyme helps support and improve cellular function (via improved mitochondrial function). It also helps prevent free-radical damage to cell mitochondria, which can cause age-related decline in egg quality (Bentov and Casper 2013). COQ10 has also been shown to improve almost all sperm parameters, including density, motility, and morphology (Safarinejad 2012). A standard dosage is 100 – 200 mg a day, but your health care provider may prescribe 500 mg a day or more as needed.

Mitochondrial function declines with age (Shigenaga et al. 1994) and structural damage to mitochondria is found more often in older women (Tatone et al. 2008) and older eggs (Wilding et al. 2001). Research has shown that adenosine triphosphate (ATP), the energy of the cell, is essential for egg maturation and development into an embryo (Van Blerkom et al. 1995). Having mitochondria packed with ATP energy seems to be key for egg quality since an egg needs energy to do all the genetic work of separating and matching chromosomes at ovulation and fertilization (Dumollard et al. 2009). Research has shown human embryos with poorly functioning mitochondria have a higher chance of disrupted chromosome processing (Wilding et al. 2003). The theory suggests that if we can help the cell replace its energy by taking CoQ10 supplements, we can improve egg function at ovulation and fertilization and have embryos with correct chromosome count (and successful pregnancies).

A recently published study in mouse models showed that aging female mouse oocytes are accompanied by mitochondrial dysfunction associated with increased oxidative stress and reduced ATP energy levels (Ben-Meir et al. 2015). The authors state that this age-related decline in egg quality could be reversed with CoQ10 supplementation (Ben-Meir et al. 2015). Another study found that adding CoQ10 to animal eggs and embryos developing in the lab increased the amount of ATP in the cells and the number of embryos developing to the blastocyst stage (day 5 after ovulation) (Stojkovc et al. 1999).

Studies with COQ10 supplements for humans undergoing IVF are limited. One study examines CoQ10 supplementation and oocyte aneuploidy (abnormality) in women undergoing IVF (Bentov et al. 2014). This double blind, placebo-controlled trial included 39 women aged 35-43 years old undergoing IVF for various reasons – half received 600 mg of CoQ10 and half received a placebo pill. 46.5% of the eggs in the CoQ10 group were abnormal, compared to 62.8% in the placebo (non-CoQ10) group. The pregnancy rate was 33% in the CoQ10 group and 26.7% in the placebo group. These differences were not significant, but the authors argue that this study lacked the power (adequate number of patients) to show a true difference in outcomes between groups.

Although definitive studies in humans have yet to prove improved egg quality and function through the use of supplemental CoQ10, there is biological plausibility of its benefit, relatively low risk of taking the supplement, and we both consider it as a recommendation when reviewing options with our patients.

> ❑ **Food Sources of CoQ10**: CoQ10 can be found in meat and poultry, although these sources most likely will not supply enough CoQ10 to make a difference to fertility unless eaten in large quantities (Bhagavan and Chopra 2006).
> ❑ **Tips for CoQ10 Supplementation**: Consider taking CoQ10 with breakfast. Taking it with a meal may increase absorption and you may experience an energy boost (which is better when you are starting your day than when you are trying to go to sleep). When taking CoQ10 supplements, please note that there are two different forms: ubiquinone and ubiquinol. Ubiquinone is not easily absorbed, and must be converted into the active form of CoQ10 called ubiquinol. Ubiquinol is the active form of CoQ10 and easily absorbed. It's best to review the dose with your medical provider, but it is usually recommended at 100-200 mg every day (although MDs regularly prescribe it at 500-600 mg per day).
> ❑ **Potential Side Effects**: Too much CoQ10 may result in gastrointestinal issues with some people.

DHEA

DHEA or dehydroepiandrosterone is a natural hormone precursor that gets converted to estrogen and testosterone in the adrenal glands and ovaries. DHEA levels decrease with age (Harper et al. 1999), and its replacement in the form of a supplement may have anti-aging effects, relieve menopause symptoms, and boost athletic performance as an alternative to anabolic steroids (Arlt 2004). DHEA's use in fertility is controversial—some providers encourage the use of DHEA especially in women with diminished ovarian reserve as a way to improve egg quantity and quality and other providers do not support its use due to lack of consistent evidence for these claims, along with its potential side effects, which we will discuss below.

The evidence for DHEA use in women with diminished ovarian reserve is mixed. An early study from Baylor University showed an increase in egg numbers in five women taking DHEA for two months (Casson et al. 2000). Another study with 25 women showed higher egg and embryo number in the women's second IVF cycle compared to their first cycle after taking DHEA (Barad and Gleicher 2006). A follow up study showed a higher pregnancy rate (28%) in patients taking DHEA for four months before an IVF cycle compared to a 10% pregnancy rate in women not taking DHEA (Barad et al. 2007).

One study showed a potential link between DHEA and chromosome function. Researchers compared a group of patients undergoing IVF with chromosomal screening of their embryos who were taking DHEA supplements to a group of patients undergoing the same treatment with IVF who were not taking DHEA. The researchers found that 61% of the embryos from the group not taking DHEA were abnormal compared to 38% abnormal embryos in the patients taking DHEA (Gleicher et al. 2010).

The controversy around DHEA includes concerns around the current evidence and potential side effects of DHEA supplementation. Reviews of the evidence regarding use of DHEA in fertility conclude that the use of DHEA should still be considered experimental and not widely recommended until further studies can be conducted (Urman and Yakin 2012). Some argue that the studies showing positive results with DHEA are too small and poorly designed to show conclusive evidence of its benefits.

DHEA is a precursor to hormones and may have significant side effects for women taking it. DHEA may be converted to testosterone and high levels of testosterone may result in oily skin, acne, hair loss, and male pattern hair growth (facial hair) in women. Other side effects linked to DHEA include impaired insulin sensitivity, impaired glucose tolerance, liver problems, and manic episodes (Yakin and Urman 2011). At least one group using DHEA for their fertility patients have reported no significant side effects in their patients (Gleicher and Barad 2011).

A recent study states that the "review of the previously published studies does not provide clear evidence that DHEA can be a useful treatment to improve ovarian function in poor responders" (Lin et al. 2015).

DHEA—Use with caution. At the time of this publication, neither of us routinely prescribe DHEA for our patients due to our concerns over the potential side effects, although we are following the evidence closely. DHEA may be considered by some fertility specialists on a case-by-case basis and there has been a lot of discussion about it, so we wanted to include it here. When DHEA is used for fertility, most studies suggest using micronized DHEA at a dose of 25 mg three times a day.

Antioxidants

Antioxidants like vitamin C, vitamin E, alpha lipoic acid, N-acetylcysteine, and melatonin are molecules that decrease oxidative stress in the body. Oxidative stress results from a buildup of free radicals or reactive oxygen molecules that are natural byproducts of metabolism within cells. These excess free radicals cause damage to DNA and mitochondria in cells. Antioxidants can neutralize these free radicals and thus decrease the damage from free radicals within cells. Some research suggests that taking antioxidants as supplements can improve egg quality by decreasing damage to DNA and mitochondria within eggs.

Eggs from older women have more oxidizing molecules and free radicals (Shigenaga et al. 1994). Women with unexplained infertility have been found to have higher than expected levels of reactive oxygen molecules (Polak et al. 2001). In mouse models, oxidative stress in eggs decreased energy production and destabilized chromosome processing (Zhang et al. 2006). Studies in women have conflicting results. One study showed women with higher antioxidant levels had a greater chance of success with IVF (Ozatik et al. 2013) while another review of multiple studies showed no good quality evidence that antioxidant supplements increase live birth rates (Showell et al. 2013).

Vitamin C (ascorbic acid) is a water-soluble antioxidant that acts as a cofactor to several enzyme reactions and metabolic pathways within cells. Vitamin C is found in ovarian follicles and thought to assist in follicular development (Luck et al. 1995), and one study showed a shorter time to pregnancy in women taking vitamin C supplements (Ruder et al. 2014).

❏ **Food Sources of Vitamin C**: Natural sources of vitamin C include oranges, guava, black currants, liver, Brussels sprouts, and broccoli.

- ❏ **Tips for Vitamin C Supplementation**: The North American Dietary Reference Intake recommends 90 mg per day and no more than 2000 mg per day for adults. Some centers recommend 500 mg daily for a potential fertility benefit (Fett 2014).
- ❏ **Potential Side Effects**: Too much vitamin C can result in indigestion, diarrhea, vomiting, flushing, headache, and disrupted sleep (WHO toxicological evaluation 2009).

Vitamin E is a fat-soluble antioxidant important in enzyme functions, gene expression, and neurologic functions. One study showed high doses of vitamin E reduced free radicals in follicular fluid (Tamura et al. 2008). Another study showed shorter time to pregnancy in women over age 35 taking supplemental vitamin E (Ruder et al. 2014).

- ❏ **Food Sources of Vitamin E**: Natural sources of vitamin E include sunflower seeds, almonds, spinach, and avocado.
- ❏ **Tips for Vitamin E Supplementation**: Recommended doses of vitamin E supplements for fertility vary from 200-600 IU daily. More is not necessarily better or safe, and the upper limit for a daily vitamin E dose should not exceed 1000 IU.
- ❏ **Potential Side Effects**: Vitamin E toxicity can include skin irritation, gastrointestinal issues, headache, and fatigue. Vitamin E can act like an anticoagulant and increase the risk of bleeding, especially in patients taking aspirin or other anticoagulants (like heparin).

Alpha lipoic acid is both fat and water soluble. It is an antioxidant found within mitochondria, where it assists with energy production (Packer et al. 1995). Some laboratory evidence suggests that alpha lipoic acid can improve egg maturation and embryo viability (Zembron-Lacny et al. 2009), but large studies are lacking.

- ❏ **Food Sources of Alpha Lipoic Acid**: Natural sources of alpha lipoic acid include spinach, liver, broccoli, and yeast.
- ❏ **Tips for Alpha Lipoic Acid Supplementation**: Supplements come in several forms, but the R-alpha lipoic acid form is more easily absorbed. A common supplemental dose is 600 mg per day.

> ❏ **Potential Side Effects**: Too much alpha lipoic acid can result in side effects such as skin tingling sensations, headache, and muscle cramps. This supplement may interfere with thyroid function and alter blood sugar levels, so patients with thyroid issues, diabetes or insulin resistance should definitely review with their medical provider before taking it.

N-acetylcysteine (NAC) is an amino acid derivative that acts as an antioxidant. It can be used as an antidote to acetaminophen overdose. N-acetylcysteine has been studied in patients with polycystic ovarian syndrome (PCOS) and found to improve ovulation (Nasr 2010) and decrease insulin and testosterone levels in these patients (Kilic-Okaman and Kucuk 2004). Other studies have shown a decrease in miscarriage rates in women taking NAC, especially in patients with PCOS (Nasr 2010 and Amin et al. 2008). Studies in animal models have shown that N-acetylcysteine reduces oxidative stress, chromosomal damage, and improves egg quality (Liu et al. 2002).

> ❏ **Food Sources of N-acetylcysteine**: N-acetylcysteine is not found naturally in foods but NAC converts into cysteine which is found in animal protein (including fish and poultry), dairy, and eggs. Vegetarian sources include soy, nuts, seeds, quinoa, broccoli, bell peppers, onion, and garlic.
> ❏ **Tips for N-acetylcysteine Supplementation**: There is no common dose for NAC supplements—studies have used doses from 600-1200 mg per day in patients.
> ❏ **Potential Side Effects**: Side effects include nausea, vomiting, and rash, and patients with asthma have reported severe allergic reactions.

Melatonin is a hormone secreted by the pineal gland at night to help regulate circadian rhythms. Melatonin is most often used as a sleep aid, but it is also an antioxidant. High levels of melatonin have been found in developed follicles with mature eggs and it may have a role in ovulation (Tamura et al. 2012). Its role in fertility is unclear, but melatonin is a powerful antioxidant that decreases oxidative damage from free radicals (Poeggeler et al. 1993). In animal studies, melatonin added to culture media reduced oxidative stress in eggs

(Jahnke et al. 1999) and increased blastocyst formation rate, which is the embryo stage on day 5-6 after ovulation that many embryos never reach (Ishizuka et al. 2000). Studies in humans undergoing IVF have compared patients' failed IVF cycles to a subsequent cycle with melatonin supplements and found an increased rate of fertilization, higher quality embryos, and a 20% higher pregnancy rate (Tamura et al. 2008 and Tamura et al. 2012).

> ❏ **Food Sources of Melatonin:** You can increase your melatonin by eating tart cherries (especially Montmorency cherries), tomatoes, asparagus, and walnuts.
> ❏ **Tips for Melatonin Supplementation:** Supplemental melatonin can disrupt natural ovulation and should not be taken while trying to conceive naturally. The dose used in women undergoing IVF is usually 3 mg at night.
> ❏ **Potential Side Effects:** Side effects may include drowsiness, dizziness, irritability, and depression.

What to Avoid: BPA, Phthalates, and other Toxins

When considering the best ways to improve egg quality and genetic function of the egg, you must also take into account the things that may harm genetic function. Most of us are aware that chemotherapy and radiation for cancer treatment can diminish reproductive potential and make women and men sterile, so it should not be too much of a stretch to consider other environmental toxins that may affect fertility on a subtler level. Two of these toxins that can be found in everyday household items are BPAs and phthalates.

BPA

BPA (bisphenol A) is a carbon-based synthetic compound that has been in commercial use since around 1957. BPA is used in many plastics and epoxy resins and can be found in everyday items such as water bottles, lining for canned food, and paper receipts. BPA has been labeled an 'endocrine disruptor' since it has been shown to bind to hormone receptors and interfere with the function of hormones like estrogen and testosterone (Kitamura et al. 2005; Welshons et al. 2006). It is estimated that up to 95% of residents in the United States would test positive for some amount of BPA in the bloodstream (Stahlhut et al. 2009; Vandenberg et al. 2012).

High levels of BPA in women have been associated with lower success with IVF (Lamb et al. 2008; Fujimoto et al. 2011) and a higher risk of miscarriage (Lathi et al. 2014). In mouse models, researchers have shown that a low dose of BPA can interfere with the final stages of egg development, leading to chromosomal imbalances in the eggs (Hunt et al. 2003).

Evidence supports the negative impact of BPA on reproduction, and until manufacturers stop using it, consumers have to take steps to actively avoid BPA. BPA is harmful all around, and should especially be avoided if you are trying to conceive or are pregnant. In animal studies, BPA has been found in amniotic fluid (Takahashi and Oishi 2000), and high levels of BPA exposure to the fetus may result in negative effects on the development of the brain and reproductive system (Cabaton et al. 2011; Tian et al. 2010).

A review of BPA and fertility research that was published in October 2014 shows that almost all aspects of fertility are affected by BPA, from development of the eggs and sperm to implantation and embryo quality (Machtinger and Orvieto 2014). Further studies are implicating BPA and other industrial chemicals as one potential causative factor in the development of polycystic ovary syndrome (PCOS) in women (Paulioura and Diamanti-Kandarakis 2013) and that mothers exposed to BPA during pregnancy increase a female child's likelihood of having PCOS later in life (Rutkowska and Rachoń 2014).

What can you do to reduce your BPA exposure?
- ❏ Eliminate plastic from your kitchen and use alternatives like glass and stainless steel. BPA can leach from plastic containers exposed to heat and detergent (dishwashers, microwaves). Many plastics state that they are "BPA free," but it may be safest to avoid plastic altogether if possible, especially since BPA free plastics often have other toxins such as phthalates in them.
- ❏ If you do use plastic, avoid polycarbonate (labeled with a '7'), which is found in many hard, reusable plastic containers.
- ❏ If you do use plastic, keep it away from heat. Do not put it in a dishwasher or microwave.

❑ Decrease take-out foods and bring your own to-go container to restaurants for leftovers as many take-out containers are full of BPA.

❑ Think about other sources of plastic in your kitchen—hot water running through a plastic-lined automatic coffee machine could be replaced with a French press or glass, pour-over coffee system.

❑ Avoid canned food, or at least get canned food that is labeled BPA free.

❑ Avoid handling paper receipts and other thermal paper (like airline and concert tickets) whenever possible. Fortunately, we live in the digital age and can have some receipts and tickets emailed to us instead of printed out.

Phthalates

Phthalates are chemicals found in commonly used products such as perfume and nail polish. Phthalates have been associated with hormone disruption and negative effects on reproduction, and animal studies have shown that phthalate exposure has a negative effect on egg development and fertilization (Dalman et al. 2008). Phthalate exposure in pregnancy has been associated with increased risk of miscarriage (Toft et al. 2012), preterm birth (Meeker et al. 2009), and reproductive development in boys (Swan et al. 2005).

Phthalates are in many cosmetic products, especially those with fragrance or strong odor. Unfortunately, manufacturers do not always list phthalate in the ingredients list (and it is often disguised as "fragrance").

What can you do to reduce your phthalate exposure?
❑ Head to your bathroom and look through all cosmetics, lotions, shampoos, nail polish, etc. and eliminate any with phthalate listed as an ingredient.

❑ Consider eliminating air fresheners and perfume.

❑ Switch to fragrance-free laundry detergent, fabric softeners, and cleaning supplies, or at least those made without phthalates.

❑ Stop using nail polish or at least use one that does not have phthalates (beware that some nail polishes listed as 'three free,'

meaning free of phthalates, formaldehyde, and toluene, actually have those ingredients).
- ❏ Phthalates are in PVC (polyvinylchloride) also known as vinyl (think shower curtains, soft plastic containers, and bags).
- ❏ Limit exposure to prepared and processed food packaged in plastic wrap.

Other toxins

A good resource for chemicals to avoid and cosmetics that are less toxic than others is the Environmental Working Group, an environmental organization founded in 1993. This group has information regarding chemicals in products on their website www.ewg.org and they have user-friendly apps that can help you navigate through products to find the least toxic one.

It's easy to get overwhelmed when you realize how many BPAs, phthalates, and other toxins are out there, but do not be too alarmed. You cannot eliminate exposure to all toxins, but you can be more aware of what you are using and make smart choices for your overall health (even when you are not trying to conceive).

What about sperm?

Male factor infertility can affect couples more than you may think. Depending on how you define male factor infertility (sperm counts or abnormalities), up to 50% of couples struggling to conceive may have a contributing sperm issue (Esteves and Agarwal 2011). Just like eggs, sperm are created through biological processes involving DNA replication, mitochondria, and ATP. Although the majority of evidence regarding supplements and reproduction focus on eggs, there are some studies that show improvements in sperm parameters and function with the use of supplements.

Men often ask how they can improve sperm counts, and Western medicine is limited. One common mistake I see is well-meaning providers prescribing testosterone for men to improve counts. But testosterone will shut down sperm production and is being investigated as a male form of contraception. It can take months for the sperm count to recover after men take testosterone, and I am too often the person explaining this to

What can men do?

- ❑ **Take antioxidants**. Antioxidants should theoretically decrease oxidative stress in sperm production. One study showed that men taking antioxidants had a higher chance of conception over time (Showell et al. 2014). Another study compared success rates with IVF treatment in the same couples with male factor infertility before and after the men took vitamin E and vitamin C daily for two months and found a significantly higher clinical pregnancy rate (Greco et al. 2005).

At our clinic, the "multivitamin" that we give to men is an antioxidant formulation because antioxidants are so important to sperm production. —Stephanie

- ❑ **Take CoQ10**. CoQ10 has been investigated as a treatment for male factor infertility, and one study showed lower CoQ10 levels in men with poor sperm parameters (Mancini et al. 1994). Several studies show that men with poor sperm parameters have significant improvements in sperm count, motility, and morphology when taking CoQ10 (Lafuente et al. 2013).
- ❑ **Take zinc**. Some men may need extra zinc, which is necessary for sperm production and testosterone metabolism—and which is lacking in most diets (Wong et al. 2002). Men may need 30mg a day of zinc whereas most multivitamins contain only 15mg.
- ❑ **Avoid toxins**. Sperm seem to be very sensitive to environmental toxins. Men with high levels of phthalates have higher incidence of infertility (Buck Louis et al. 2014), and high levels of BPA in men are associated with lower sperm counts (Knez et al. 2014).
- ❑ **Get a check up**. Medical issues such as varicoceles (an enlargement of the veins within the scrotum), diabetes, infections, and other chronic diseases can negatively affect sperm production.

❏ **Get a semen analysis**. Men may be reluctant to get a sperm analysis since many of them assume that if sexual function is adequate and they have an ejaculate that they must have sperm, but this is not always the case. It is estimated that 1% of the population has azoospermia (no sperm in the ejaculate) and the incidence may be much higher in the infertility population (Gudeloglu and Parekattil 2013).

Egg quality is a relatively new field of study in the western world, but the research is showing what Chinese medicine has known for a long time—that taking steps to improve your health and avoiding harmful substances may increase your fertility and possibly your egg and sperm quality as well. In the next chapter, we'll talk about timing your cycle to optimize natural conception.

5

Optimizing Natural Conception

If you've been trying unsuccessfully to get pregnant and it's been months since you've stopped using birth control, it's time to learn more about your body, the menstrual cycle, and ways to optimize natural conception.

In the United States, most of us don't learn how to get pregnant—we learn how to not get pregnant. Women often come to our offices needing to be coached on the basics, so here we go!

Although your health teacher in high school probably made it sound like getting pregnant was terrifyingly easy, human reproduction is complicated and not very efficient. Women lose hundreds (maybe thousands) of eggs each cycle and ovulate only one. Men make millions of sperm a day for that one single sperm to try to fertilize the egg. Once an egg and sperm fertilize, not every fertilized egg (now embryo) continues to develop or implant in the uterus.

Chances of Success with Each Cycle

When a couple is in their early twenties (peak fertility), for each menstrual cycle, the chances that a sperm will fertilize an egg and result in a baby nine months later is approximately 25%. As the eggs and sperm age, fewer of them can complete all the genetic changes needed to fertilize and continue developing into a healthy embryo. When a couple is in their 40s, the chances of live birth with a single menstrual cycle and natural conception are approximately 5%. This is why starting a family later in life can take longer than we think, or want.

> *Most patients are very surprised and disappointed when I explain the chances of success for natural conception leading to a baby with each cycle. But I share this with patients in a positive light so that they'll have realistic expectations—and as a way to explain that, although frustrating, it is actually "normal" to take time to conceive.*
> *—Lora*

The Menstrual Cycle, Ovulation, and Timing of Conception

A menstrual cycle starts and ends with the first day of bleeding from month to month. A typical menstrual cycle is approximately 28 days, with ovulation occurring on cycle day (CD) 14. A menstrual period should begin on what would have been CD 29.

According to TCM, a woman should have a cycle that starts with red blood and a moderate flow that continues for 3 – 7 days without clots or cramps. Both pre- and post-ovulation should be 14 days, with a little more variance allowed in the pre-ovulation phase. The post-ovulation (or luteal phase) should be 12 – 14 days.

Using Ovulation Predictor Kits (OPKs) and charting your Basal Body Temperature (BBT) can help you track different aspects of your menstrual cycle. We'll explain how to use these tools later on in this chapter, but basically, OPKs will tell you when you are going to ovulate and charting your BBT will tell you if you ovulate and what your cycle is doing outside ovulation time.

> *"I had no idea that I wasn't ovulating…" —Lisa, Acupuncture patient*

Another thing OPKs and BBT charting will help you find out is if you have a classic "normal" cycle. If your cycle deviates from the norm, it doesn't mean that you cannot get pregnant, but the 'normal' cycle is a template for which we are always striving.

When Should We Be Trying?

One important aspect of optimizing natural conception is timing intercourse. None of us wants to have to schedule our intimate time with our partners, but when you have been struggling to conceive, you often need to plan sex. Think of the woman's egg as a ship at port and the sperm as the passengers. Once that ship has set sail, there is no more chance to get on board that cycle!

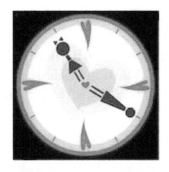

While intimacy on a schedule is less than ideal and can be stressful for a couple, learning more about the cycle and tools that reveal optimal times to try can decrease the stress people put on themselves to 'time it right.'

We've both had patients come in who just had the timing wrong. Once that was addressed, many of these patients went on to get pregnant easily.

> *"We didn't even know that we were having sex too late in my cycle."—Sarah, Acupuncture patient*

Cervical Fluid and Your Peak Day

The most fertile time in a woman's cycle is the last day of the most fertile cervical fluid, or the 'peak day.' Your peak day generally occurs one or two days prior to ovulation. Fertile cervical fluid should look like uncooked egg-white (clear and slippery). If you don't observe 'egg-white' cervical fluid, then your most fertile day is the last day of the wettest cervical fluid you observe.

Cervical fluid contains sugars that help nourish the sperm and estrogen that acts on the fluid to help transport the sperm to the woman's reproductive system (Fordney-Settlage 1981).

> *At our clinic, we advise couples as to the frequency of intercourse pre-ovulation, depending on the health of the man's sperm. Prior to fertile cervical fluid, we recommend intercourse every other day starting five days prior to ovulation. When cervical fluid arrives, then if the man has a normal sperm count (over 20 million per ml), intercourse can be daily through the day when his partner's temperature rises. If the man has a low sperm count (under 20 million per ml), it is optimal to have*

Sperm can be found swimming and able to fertilize an egg for up to four days in the woman's reproductive system while the egg can only able be fertilized for 12 – 24 hours after it is released from the follicle in the ovary. The goal of timing intercourse is to have sperm ready and waiting for the egg when you ovulate, so the best time to have intercourse is the week prior to projected ovulation and coinciding with the days of fertile cervical fluid.

Ovulation Predictor Kits (OPKs)

Ovulation predictor kits (OPKs) are used to predict ovulation (release of the egg from the ovary). They come in many forms, including sticks used prior to ovulation that measure hormones in the urine to fertility monitors that monitor you all cycle long. The urine sticks come in midstream sticks (that you hold in your urine stream) to dip sticks (that you dip in a cup). The midstream sticks tend to be more sensitive and easier to use, but they are also more expensive.

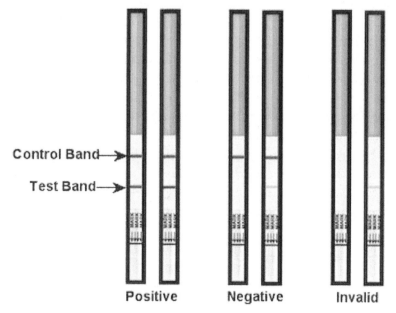

OPKs monitor the luteinizing hormone (LH) in your urine. LH is a gonadotropin hormone released from the pituitary gland under the brain that signals the release of the egg from the ovary. As the primary follicle matures in the ovary it produces rising levels of estrogen that signal the pituitary gland to release LH. The LH rises before the egg is released from the ovary. This communication of hormones is one of the many variables that need to be in balance for conception to occur.

Ovulation happens approximately 36 hours after your first positive OPK test. The LH may remain high for 12 – 36 hours. Once you have a positive OPK in the middle of your cycle, you do not need to keep testing.

Start checking OPKs one week prior to when you think that you ovulate. If you do not know when you should start testing, count back 21 days from the length of the shortest cycle that you have had. For example, if historically your shortest cycle was 26 days, then you would start doing OPKs on cycle day 5. If you have a 35 day cycle, you would start using the OPKs on CD 14. Test daily until you get a positive OPK. You only need to use OPKs until you know that you ovulate and when you ovulate. This usually takes a few cycles of monitoring.

> *Timing intercourse can be frustrating and stressful for couples trying to conceive. Once I explain the physiology around ovulation and fertilization, couples can hopefully relax a little again. The timing of intercourse is not a precise science, and I am amazed at some of the "friendly" advice my patients get from well-meaning family and friends about it. Sperm is viable (able to fertilize and swim) for 48 – 96 hours, depending on a lot of variables, and the egg is viable (able to be fertilized) for 12 – 24 hours. I recommend couples have intercourse 2 – 3 times surrounding ovulation and to start before ovulation—not wait for a positive OPK test since they sometimes do not work and patients can miss a cycle if they wait too long. However, if patients can only have sex once in the whole cycle, then I recommend having intercourse when the OPK is positive (about 24 – 36 hours before the egg is released). That way, the sperm is there and ready when the egg arrives. —Lora*

Basal Body Temperature (BBT)

Another tool that aids in understanding your menstrual cycle in order to increase your chances of pregnancy is the BBT chart. BBT charts are not for predicting ovulation, but rather to show if you are ovulating, when you ovulated, and other temperature patterns that will be helpful for you and your fertility acupuncturist. Taking your BBT at the same time every morning may seem like a hassle, but the insight into your cycle that you and your acupuncturist gain makes it well worth the effort.

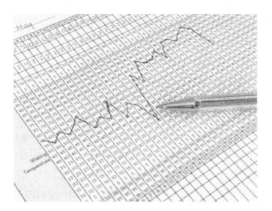

If you are thinking about getting pregnant, it is good to start charting your BBT right away. Taking your BBT shows patterns in your cycle, and it usually takes about 3 months or 3 cycles to see those patterns emerge. But once they do, you should be able to detect:
❏ A short or long follicular (pre-ovulation) phase
❏ An ovulation with a weak temperature spike
❏ A short luteal (post-ovulation) phase
❏ A luteal phase temperature that is slow to rise or quick to fall

> *"Once I started charting, I finally understood why we hadn't gotten pregnant."*
> *–Tammy, Acupuncture Patient*

How Do I Take My BBT?
❏ Take your temperature each day first thing after you wake up—before getting up or engaging in any other activity and after at least three hours of consecutive sleep.
❏ Use a thermometer that is accurate to at least 1/10th of a degree. A thermometer with memory recall is helpful if you wake up, know that you are not going to get three more hours of consecutive sleep, and need to take your temperature before you want to go back to sleep.
❏ If you are using a digital thermometer, wait until it beeps before checking the temperature, usually about a minute. If you are using a

glass basal thermometer, you will need to wait longer, about five minutes.

❑ Set a target time to take your temperature and try to take it at the same time every day.

❑ If you cannot take your temperature at the same time every day, you will need to adjust the temperature. If you get up later, it is warmer out and so are you, and you will need to decrease the temperature to match your target time.

    ❑ For every half hour later than your target time, decrease the temperature by 0.1 degrees Fahrenheit.

    ❑ If you take your temperature a half hour earlier than your target time, increase the temperature by 0.1 degrees Fahrenheit from your normal time.

❑ If the temperature falls between two numbers on a glass thermometer, always record the lower temperature.

❑ Keep a chart of your temperature throughout your cycle. Here's a link to a BBT chart that you can use: www.babyhopes.com/download/bbtchart.pdf

❑ Temperature patterns have meaning in TCM diagnosis and will affect how your fertility acupuncturist diagnoses and treats you. Put the adjusted temperatures on your chart daily. Record all other relevant information on your chart, such as cervical fluid, intercourse, excess stress, alcohol consumption, cramps, bloating, headaches, illness, pain, premenstrual symptoms, and so on, as these may affect your temperature and will also give additional information to your acupuncturist.

Remember: Adjust your BBT by 0.1 degree for every half hour deviation from your target time.

BBT Chart Examples: (reproduced with permission from FertilityUK.org)

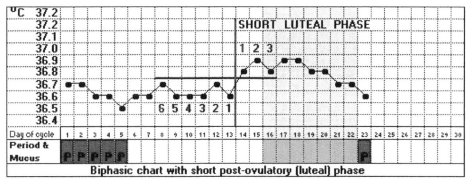

A short luteal phase, a post-ovulation that lasts less than 12 days, is often a sign of Kidney Yang Deficiency.

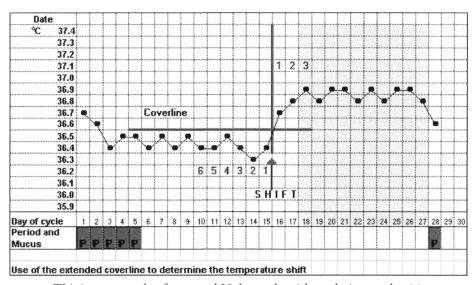

This is an example of a normal 28 day cycle with ovulation on day 14.

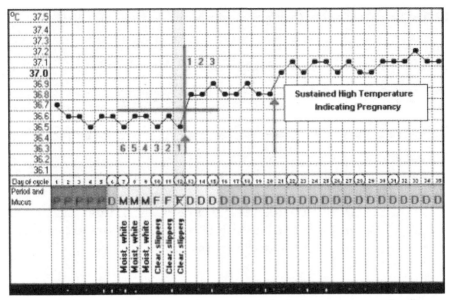

This is an example of a pregnancy chart and is called tri-phasic, meaning that there are three distinct temperature levels – pre-ovulation, post-ovulation and then the temperature rises again when there is a pregnancy.

Successful conception is a delicate process with many variables, but TCM can help optimize your overall health so you and your body are ready!

6

Your First Acupuncture Treatment

When people make their first appointment to see an acupuncturist, they are often surprised at the length of both the initial appointment (usually about 90 minutes long) and the intake form (usually about 5 – 7 pages long). They often wonder why their acupuncturist cares about their childhood, their likes and dislikes, and their sleep habits.

The typical acupuncture intake form covers everything from physical to emotional health history, what you eat, how you spend your time, and the status of your relationships. Each aspect of your life is important to your acupuncturist because all of these things affect the health of your body.

The Interview and Examination

When you come in for the first time, your visit will begin with an extensive interview covering most aspects of your health and fertility history. Your acupuncturist will then examine your tongue and feel your pulses. All of the information gathered will be assessed to create a total picture of your state of health.

Because Chinese medicine evolved in a time before modern diagnostics, such as blood work and MRIs, the acupuncturist uses signs on the tongue and the rhythm and strength of pulses to gain insight into the health of the internal organ systems and the patient's state of overall health. This method of diagnosis is subtler and allows the acupuncturist to find emerging patterns of illness rather than problems that already exist. For example, a swollen tongue indicates fluid retention, a pale tongue indicates deficiency in blood, and a red tongue shows excess heat.

Your acupuncturist will feel your pulse in three separate positions and at three different depths, as each position corresponds to a different organ system. They will look for different qualities in the pulse, such as excess or deficiency. A big pulse, for example, indicates excess heat while a weak pulse shows deficiency. A pulse that feels like a dolphin cresting under the fingers means an excess in dampness. These are just a few examples in a subtle and comprehensive diagnostic system that has been refined over the millennia.

Both Western and Eastern medicine have powerful tools for looking inside the body and evaluating your fertility, so be sure to review any tests you have from your Western medicine provider with your acupuncturist. Western medicine uses blood tests, semen analyses, ultrasounds, and hysterosalpingograms (test for fallopian tube patency). Chinese medicine uses the constitutional diagnosis to see how fertile the patient is and what might be blocking that fertility. Together, these diagnostics create a powerful picture of one's fertility.

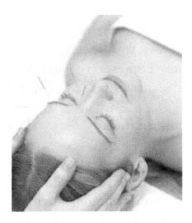

The Acupuncture Treatment

> *"I was so worried about the acupuncture needles and then I didn't even feel them go in!"*
> *—Patricia, acupuncture patient*

The next step, as your acupuncturist begins to address your imbalances, is the acupuncture treatment itself.

The acupuncture treatment itself lasts approximately 30 minutes and is usually very relaxing—most patients find it restorative. The patient is placed in a relaxed position, either face up or face down, and thin, disposable, sterile needles are placed in acupuncture points on Qi pathways (called meridians) to help the flow of Qi throughout the body.

Even when working on a reproductive issue, the needles are not placed into the reproductive organ areas! Most of the points are located from the elbows down, the knees down and on the back and the abdomen above the pubic bone. Normally, patients do not even feel the needles going in and some even fall asleep on the table.

Most acupuncturists recommend treatment approximately once a week, but the frequency and timing in the cycle are determined by your personal situation. If you are receiving Western fertility treatments in conjunction with acupuncture treatments, be sure to communicate your medications and timing of important treatments like inseminations and embryo transfers to your acupuncturist.

At the end of your visit to the fertility acupuncturist, you will get a treatment plan customized especially for you. It will cover all aspects of your fertility and overall health. You will be given recommendations on frequency of acupuncture and on appropriate supplements, nutrition, lifestyle choices, and possibly a customized Chinese herbal medicine formula.

> *"After my first visit to the fertility acupuncturist, I relaxed, knowing that I had an advocate with me on my fertility journey. I had hope again." —Gretchen, acupuncture patient*

By the end of your visit with your acupuncturist, you should feel like you have taken a positive step in doing everything you can to get you closer to your dream of having a child.

Fertility Acupuncturist as Guide

One area where fertility acupuncturists can be very helpful is in their ability to help you navigate the sometimes complicated world of Western fertility treatments (if you find yourself there). Your fertility acupuncturist may know the fertility doctors, what they have to offer (in terms of diagnostics and treatment) and what you can expect.

> *At our clinic, we understand the place Western medicine has in the diagnosis and treatment of infertility. We often refer to reproductive endocrinologists for testing and, when appropriate, treatment. —Stephanie*

Good fertility acupuncturists are really much more than great TCM practitioners (although that is a key quality); they can also be a guide who will have the time to discuss your options and help you choose the fertility paths that are best for you.

7

Assisted Reproductive Technology: The Western Approach to Fertility Treatment

Western medicine has adopted Assisted Reproductive Technology (ART) as the primary means for helping a couple conceive. These methods use artificial or partially artificial means such as ovarian stimulation medications, intrauterine insemination, and in vitro fertilization to aid in conception.

While some people focus primarily on ART methods to aid in conception, others use these methods as a complement to Eastern medicine fertility techniques. As you will see in the next chapter, TCM and ART work very well together, and each method often increases the success rate of the other.

If you are looking into ART, this chapter will help you understand your options.

Western Medicine Evaluation: What to Expect

Infertility is defined as the inability to conceive after 12 months of trying. Most providers will recommend a fertility evaluation in any woman who has not conceived within a year of trying and will often encourage an evaluation earlier in women over the age of 35 who have not conceived after six months of trying. The evaluation will include a detailed medical history and a physical exam, as well as several tests, which are detailed below.

In the evaluation, the provider will review the patient's medical history in detail, including their medications, chronic illnesses, and surgeries. They will ask about pregnancy history and menstrual history (including regularity of cycles). If there is a male partner, he should attend the first visit because his health history is important to the evaluation as well.

The results of this evaluation will not only shed light on why a woman or couple may be having trouble conceiving but will also guide which treatment options are ideal for that particular woman/couple.

Common Tests in a Western Fertility Evaluation

Western fertility testing includes blood work and anatomy evaluations for the female partner and a semen analysis for the male partner. After initial testing results are reviewed, additional testing may be advised.

Blood work includes an evaluation of the hormones that are essential for reproductive health and of the ovarian reserve, which is a term used to describe the capacity of the ovaries to produce fertilizable eggs and the quality of those oocytes as gleaned by testing AMH, FSH and antral follicle count (these tests are described below).

A complete anatomy evaluation includes an ultrasound to evaluate ovarian health and uterine shape as well as a hysterosalpingogram (HSG) to evaluate the openness of the fallopian tubes and the integrity of the uterine cavity (inside the uterine wall where the embryo implants).

Anatomy testing

- ❏ **Pelvic ultrasound**: A transvaginal ultrasound to examine the female reproductive organs. This ultrasound can help diagnose problems in the uterus and the ovaries, like fibroids and ovarian cysts. It can also help the provider determine your ovarian reserve by looking at your antral follicle count (see discussion below under egg health/supply).
- ❏ **Hysterosalpingogram** (HSG): A test that can show whether the fallopian tubes are open or not. During this test, a small catheter is placed in the cervix and contrast liquid is placed through this tube into the uterine cavity. Fluoroscopy (small doses of X-ray images) is used to watch the contrast material flow from the uterine cavity and through both fallopian tubes. This test also provides a good assessment of the uterine cavity and can diagnose subtle issues such as uterine scarring or small polyps that can be missed on the pelvic ultrasound.

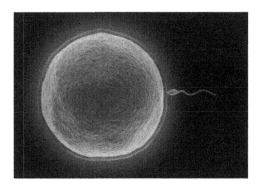

Egg/sperm health and supply

- ❏ **Antral follicle count**: Follicles are fluid-filled structures in the ovaries. Each follicle contains one egg, and the antral follicle count gives us an idea of how many follicles are present. A normal antral follicle count is approximately 10 – 15 total follicles between both ovaries. A very high antral follicle count may be associated with polycystic ovarian syndrome, and a very low antral follicle count may be associated with diminished ovarian reserve.

- ❏ **Follicle stimulating hormone (FSH) and estradiol**: These two hormones should be tested early in the cycle, usually cycle day three (the third day of menstrual bleeding). A high FSH is associated with diminished ovarian reserve. Every laboratory is slightly different, but in general, a FSH of <10 mIU/mL is considered normal. Estradiol should be checked with the FSH to ensure accuracy. A high estradiol level can falsely lower a FSH level and mask diminished ovarian reserve.

- ❏ **Anti-müllerian hormone (AMH)**: A hormone found in the ovaries. AMH is a relatively new ovarian reserve test and interpretation is still under investigation. In general, AMH is considered a quantitative assessment of ovarian reserve. A low AMH is associated with a lower response to ovarian stimulation medication (which is a type of fertility treatment).

- ❏ **Semen analysis**: Semen testing provides information on the quantity and quality of sperm parameters, which include sperm count, motility (their ability to move), morphology (their shape) and other parameters.

Please note that no blood test is going to predict pregnancy. Poor results with ovarian reserve and other testing may predict lower response to fertility treatment and lower success rates with fertility treatment, but they are not absolute predictors of pregnancy.

> *I have had many patients with extremely poor ovarian reserve testing who have conceived on their own after receiving this disappointing information. As long as someone has eggs and is ovulating, they still have the chance of conceiving.* —Lora

Other tests that may be offered

After your initial results are reviewed, your provider may want to do follow up testing depending on what they have found. These tests may include the following:

- ❏ **Thyroid function**: Hypothyroidism can be associated with an increased risk of miscarriage and other poor obstetric outcomes.
- ❏ **Prolactin**: Usually, prolactin is normal with regular menstrual cycles, but if it is elevated, it can be associated with implantation issues and miscarriage risk.
- ❏ **Rubella and varicella titers**: These tests are to confirm immunity to these two viruses (German measles and chickenpox). Being infected with these viruses while pregnant can cause miscarriage or birth defects.
- ❏ **Genetic screening options**: Blood tests to screen the couple for gene mutations that lead to preventable disease in children. (These options will be detailed later on in this chapter).

Treatment Options

ART options essentially involve ovarian stimulation with medication followed by intrauterine insemination (IUI) or in vitro fertilization (IVF). IUI is the process of washing/preparing the sperm and placing it with a catheter past the cervix into the uterus during ovulation. IVF is the process of removing eggs from the ovaries with an in-office, 15-minute procedure called an egg retrieval. The eggs are then fertilized outside the body, and the developing embryo(s) are inserted into the uterus with a catheter.

IVF is considerably more complicated and expensive than IUI. Most couples will try ovulation induction with or without IUI as a first step and consider IVF at a later time if the IUIs are not successful. Patients who should consider IVF as a first step are those with blocked fallopian tubes and/or patients with very low sperm counts.

> *When first introducing treatment options for patients, I often say: "There are a lot of bells and whistles to fertility treatment, but when we simplify it, there are really two options: low tech and high tech. The low tech options are ovulation induction with or without intrauterine insemination. The high tech option is IVF." Reminding them of these two broad options helps improve the understanding of the options from the start. We then review the details of each option and how they would benefit the patient's personal situation. —Lora*

Ovulation induction/medications

The menstrual cycle is basically divided into two phases—the follicular phase, in which one egg is selected for development and maturation, and the luteal phase, which is after ovulation when the body is preparing for embryo implantation if the egg was successfully fertilized with a sperm in that cycle.

In the follicular phase, one egg out of a set of recruitable eggs (see discussion on the antral follicle count above) is selected and ovulated through a delicate balance of hormone interaction. Ovulation induction involves giving medication in the early follicular phase (starting within the first 2 – 5 days of menses) in order to recruit more than one egg to ovulate. Releasing 2 – 3 eggs will improve the odds of pregnancy (and will also increase the risk of multiples to about 5 – 8% over the naturally occurring 1% in couples). Ovulation induction does not always result in the recruitment and release of more than one egg, yet it is still associated with a slightly higher pregnancy rate than natural conception.

Ovulation medications come in the form of pills and injections. The pills most commonly used are Clomid® (sertolene) and Femara® (letrozole). These are usually prescribed for five days at the beginning of the cycle (from cycle day 3 – 7, for example). They are anti-estrogen medications and encourage the pituitary gland to release more follicle-stimulating hormone (FSH) than it would in a natural cycle (more FSH can result in multiple egg recruitment).

> **Clomid vs. Femara.** Clomid® has been prescribed as an ovulation
> medication since the 1960s. Side effects may include multiple gestation,
> headaches, mood swings, vision changes, hot flashes, thin uterine lining,
> and ovarian cysts. While Letrozole (Femara®) is not approved by the FDA
> for use for fertility treatment, it is still widely prescribed for this use. Fewer
> side effects occur with Letrozole (Femara®) than with Clomid®, and
> patients usually tolerate it better.

The other option for ovulation induction is gonadotropin medications, such as
Follistim® and Gonal-F®. These are injectable medications given in the
beginning of the cycle to recruit multiple eggs. Unlike the oral medications
that 'trick' the body into producing more follicle-stimulating hormone (FSH),
the gonadotropins actually are FSH.

Gonadotropins are used for egg recruitment in IVF because they have a high
success rate in recruiting multiple eggs. Gonadotropins may also be used for
egg recruitment for IUI cycles. They are given as a daily injection for
approximately 7 – 12 days until the eggs are ready to ovulate. There is a higher
chance of multiples using gonadotropins compared to oral medication.

Ovulation induction is key for people who are not ovulating on their own, but
people who are ovulating regularly may still benefit from these medications, so
they are often used in conjunction with other methods of ART.

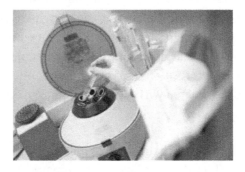

Intrauterine insemination (IUI)

Intrauterine insemination (IUI) is a common ART procedure. IUI is the
process of washing/preparing the sperm and placing it with a catheter past the

cervix into the uterine cavity during ovulation. The procedure is quick and relatively simple. For the patient, it is similar to a gynecology exam (pap smear). The whole process takes approximately five minutes.

This procedure may be beneficial in many ways, including:
- ❏ **The preparing/washing of the sperm**: This process removes any non-viable sperm as well as the acidic components in the ejaculate from prostate secretions that impede sperm motility. It also stimulates sperm activity.
- ❏ **Cervical factor infertility**: The cervix is a natural filter, and one of its jobs is to filter out the acidic components of ejaculate and allow motile sperm into the uterine cavity. But some women may have cervixes that filter too well due to decreased secretions or scar tissue. Although there is no definitive way to diagnose cervical factor infertility, the process of placing a catheter through the cervix and depositing the motile sperm into the uterine cavity bypasses this issue.
- ❏ **Timing the sperm/egg exposure**: Timing the placement of sperm in the reproductive tract around the time of the egg arriving in the fallopian tube improves the odds of conception.

Timing of the IUI may be done with either ovulation predictor kits or a transvaginal ultrasound. Ovulation predictor kits (OPKs) or fertility monitors turn positive when the pituitary gland releases a surge of luteinizing hormone, which is released from the pituitary gland to signal the final maturation and release or ovulation of the egg. OPKs are simple, but may not work for all patients and may be frustrating if they never turn positive or give false positive results.

Another option for timing IUIs is a mid-cycle transvaginal ultrasound. The maturing egg is located within a pocket of fluid within the ovary called a follicle. As the egg matures, the fluid increases such that in the middle of the cycle, a dominant follicle can be seen by transvaginal ultrasound. Once a follicle is a certain size (approximately 18 – 20 mm), the egg inside is mature. A patient may take a shot to trigger ovulation once the follicle is mature in size. This trigger shot mimics the natural LH surge and causes ovulation approximately 36 hours later. The IUI is usually done the day after the trigger shot.

If patients have regular cycles and OPKs work for them, they may consider this option for timing the IUI. The ultrasound/trigger shot option for timing IUI provides reassurance that the follicle is mature and the uterine lining is of adequate thickness. The trigger shot also encourages the ovaries to make more estrogen and progesterone in the luteal phase to help with embryo implantation.

Timing the trigger shot. The timing of the trigger shot and IUI do not have to be precise. Some patients have the impression that the sperm gets only one try with the egg, but the sperm may be viable for 48 – 96 hours and continues swimming in and out of the reproductive tract during that time. Since the egg is only viable for 12 – 24 hours, the goal is to have the sperm there waiting when the egg comes into the fallopian tube. So if a patient receives the trigger shot on a Monday, for example, she will ovulate Tuesday evening and the IUI should be done sometime during the day on Tuesday. Patients have plenty to stress about—the timing of the IUI should not be one of them.

The success of IUIs depends on the couple undergoing treatment but usually is not higher than 25% each try. Some patients ask about doing two IUIs in a cycle sequentially in an effort to improve odds of sperm exposure. This is an extra cost to patients and multiple studies show that double IUIs are no more successful than single IUIs for patients. Although IUIs help with timing, sperm stimulation, and cervical factors, they do not ensure that the egg ovulated is viable, that the sperm will fertilize the egg, or that the fallopian tubes will function correctly, which is why some patients turn to IVF.

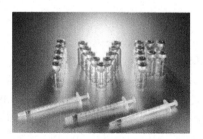

In vitro fertilization (IVF)

In vitro fertilization (IVF) has revolutionized fertility treatment since the birth of the first IVF baby in 1978. A simple way to think about IVF is that the process of conception that usually occurs within the fallopian tubes (the egg and sperm fertilizing and the first few days of embryo development) happens outside of the body in the IVF lab.

IVF was first developed for women with tubal disease as a means to bypass the fallopian tubes. The process involves retrieving the eggs out of the body, creating embryos in the IVF lab, and then replacing the embryo(s) into the uterine cavity for implantation.

IVF has expanded from patients with tubal disease to those with male factor infertility, endometriosis, unexplained infertility, and beyond. It is certainly more complicated and expensive than trying to conceive naturally or with IUIs, but it is significantly more successful.

If you are considering IVF, here are the basic steps you should expect:
- ❏ **Preparing the ovaries with birth control pills**. This step involves taking birth control pills for approximately three weeks to allow a good number of eggs to be recruited in the next step. While there are protocols for IVF without the use of birth control pills, this is the most common first step in IVF.
- ❏ **Ovarian stimulation with gonadotropins**. This step involves taking daily injections of follicle stimulating hormone (FSH) to stimulate the recruitment of multiple eggs.
- ❏ **Suppression of ovulation with an additional medication**. Lupron® or Antagonist medications are given during the cycle to prevent ovulation during egg development.
- ❏ **Egg retrieval**. A 15-minute procedure in which eggs are gently removed from the ovaries vaginally. In this procedure, a small needle is passed through the top of the vaginal wall under transvaginal ultrasound guidance into each follicle (fluid surrounding the egg). The follicular fluid is drained with gentle suction, and the egg comes with the fluid into a tube. The patient is usually given intravenous medication/conscious sedation during this procedure to keep them comfortable.
- ❏ **Fertilization**. In this step, eggs and sperm are combined with either conventional insemination or intracytoplasmic sperm

---

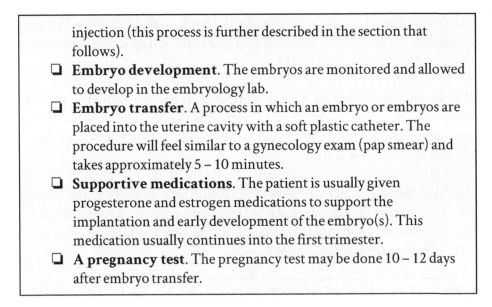

injection (this process is further described in the section that follows).

❑ **Embryo development**. The embryos are monitored and allowed to develop in the embryology lab.

❑ **Embryo transfer**. A process in which an embryo or embryos are placed into the uterine cavity with a soft plastic catheter. The procedure will feel similar to a gynecology exam (pap smear) and takes approximately 5 – 10 minutes.

❑ **Supportive medications**. The patient is usually given progesterone and estrogen medications to support the implantation and early development of the embryo(s). This medication usually continues into the first trimester.

❑ **A pregnancy test**. The pregnancy test may be done 10 – 12 days after embryo transfer.

Fertilization with IVF. There are two options for fertilization of eggs after egg retrieval: conventional insemination or intracytoplasmic sperm injection (ICSI). Conventional insemination involves placing the eggs and washed sperm together and passively waiting to see if fertilization occurs. ICSI involves the active method of fertilizing, in which one sperm is injected into one mature egg by an embryologist.

ICSI has revolutionized male factor fertility treatment and allowed men to have children who would not have been able to 30 years ago. Some IVF clinics recommend ICSI to all of their patients while others recommend it based on the patient's personal history. It is important to review both options with your provider.

Limitations of IVF. The success of IVF gets better as the technology improves, but it is never 100% successful, and the outcome depends on the patient who is undergoing treatment. IVF is especially limited by egg quality and quantity. Patients with a high number of good quality eggs/embryos will have the highest chance of success with IVF.

Society in general perpetuates the myth that IVF can overcome any fertility issue, but this is simply not true. If tabloids were true, then IVF would work for anyone who was famous or wealthy enough, but if a patient has poor quality or a low number of eggs available each cycle (diminished ovarian reserve), success rates with IVF will be low. In some cases, patients may be encouraged to explore the possibility of using donor eggs to increase their chances of conception.

IVF with Donor Egg. It is important to learn about all ART options that are available. In patients with premature ovarian failure, diminished ovarian reserve, or advanced reproductive age, IVF with donor egg(s) is a highly successful option for family building. If egg quality is the real issue in a couple trying to conceive, IVF with a donor egg can be a good alternative.

I was shopping one day at my local grocery store when a former acupuncture patient of mine—a woman who went on to use donor eggs—came up to me pushing her cart with a beautiful baby boy staring at me with big brown eyes. My patient looked at me with tears in her very blue eyes and said to me, "I am so grateful that it never worked out with my own eggs. We got the perfect child for us and we couldn't be any happier." That story has never left me. I sometimes tell this story to patients to give them hope and the courage to move on to a donor egg if they need to. —Stephanie

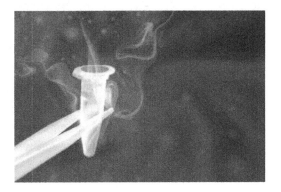

Cryopreservation and Vitrification. Cryopreservation has revolutionized the options available for fertility treatment and may also be considered a form of fertility preservation.

With cryopreservation, patients undergo all the first steps of the IVF process, but after egg retrieval, the eggs are frozen. When the patient is ready to conceive in the future, the eggs will be thawed then fertilized with sperm and the resulting embryo(s) can be transferred into the woman's uterus for implantation. Alternatively, patients who conceive with IVF may have embryos cryopreserved, which gives them the option of returning for a frozen embryo transfer for siblings in the future.

One single advancement in IVF technology within the last 10 years has revolutionized options for patients undergoing advanced ART treatments: vitrification for cryopreservation.

Freezing embryos (cryopreservation) has been available for decades, but a slow-freezing method was used and it resulted in many embryos not surviving the thawing procedure. Vitrification is a fast-freezing method that, if done by highly skilled embryologists, results in very high embryo survival rates (97% or higher) and similar or higher pregnancy rates than the rates for fresh embryo transfer. With vitrification, there has been a shift away from the assumption that frozen embryos are less successful.

One significant benefit to freezing embryos is that it allows the patient to fully recover from the IVF cycle/recruitment phase before conceiving. Ovarian stimulation of multiple eggs can result in a condition known as ovarian hyperstimulation syndrome (OHSS), in which the patient becomes bloated and uncomfortable. In women with OHSS, immediately proceeding with embryo transfer will result in worsening symptoms in the first trimester of pregnancy.

> *I am very comfortable offering cryopreservation to my patients, especially in the setting of high ovarian response to IVF treatment. In our clinic, we have found a higher pregnancy rate and less severe ovarian hyperstimulation syndrome in women who wait to transfer embryos until after their body has recovered from the IVF cycle.*
> *—Lora*

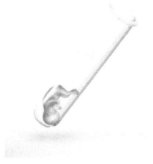

Genetic Testing and ART

Genetic testing is a broad term and may be used in several types of ART methods. There is genetic testing of patients planning to conceive and genetic testing of embryos before implantation. The different options in general are as follows:

- ❏ **Genetic testing of patients planning to conceive**. This process involves doing blood tests on both partners to see if they carry genetic mutations that may be passed on to their children. For example, a couple can be completely healthy and have no family history of cystic fibrosis, but if they both carry the same genetic mutation, their child has a 25% chance of having cystic fibrosis. If patients find out they are carriers for a genetic disease, options include early prenatal testing (for instance, an amniocentesis during pregnancy) or screening embryos for the genetic defect before implantation (via IVF).
- ❏ **Genetic testing of embryos for specific diseases**, also known as preimplantation genetic diagnosis and an example of some of the amazing advances in reproductive technology that have occurred over the last 20 years. If partners know they are carriers for a genetic disease, they have the ability to do IVF and screen the embryos for the genetic disease before implantation. They can then choose to implant an embryo without the genes for cystic fibrosis or other genetic diseases.
- ❏ **Genetic testing of embryos for chromosomal number**, also known as preimplantation genetic screening and comprehensive chromosomal screening. This testing allows us to screen embryos for

the correct number of chromosomes. The majority of embryos with an incorrect number of chromosomes are not viable, which means that if they are implanted, the result will probably be a negative pregnancy test or a miscarriage. (One exception that often does result in a live birth is Down syndrome, in which there are three copies of the number 21 chromosome).

Genetic screening of embryos has been available in one form or another for more than 20 years. As the technology has improved, its use as an embryo selection tool in IVF cycles has increased. Genetic screening is one way to keep high success rates with a lower number of embryos transferred.

Summary

Whether it's ovulation induction for patients with ovulatory dysfunction, IUI for patients with low sperm counts, or IVF for patients with more serious fertility issues, ART methods provide useful options to patients who are having difficulty conceiving.

These methods may be used alone or in conjunction with TCM methods for maximizing chances of conception. In the next chapter, we'll look at what TCM fertility enhancement looks like alongside an ART cycle.

8

TCM Fertility Enhancement for ART

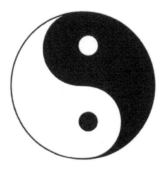

If you choose to take advantage of assisted reproductive technology (ART) in your journey to creating a family, Traditional Chinese Medicine (TCM) will remain an important part of your treatment plan.

Let's look at how TCM and ART work together. In preparation for ART, TCM is used to get both the man and the woman as healthy as possible to strengthen both eggs and sperm and get the woman prepared for pregnancy. During ART, TCM focuses on improving ART outcomes in many ways, like increasing blood flow to the reproductive organs, assisting in follicular growth, and improving sperm parameters.

There is mounting evidence that acupuncture improves ART outcomes. In February 2015, researchers published a study on using all of Chinese medicine—not just acupuncture or herbs, but also lifestyle and nutrition suggestions—to improve IVF outcomes. They found that when "whole systems" TCM was used in conjunction with IVF, it was associated with more live births and fewer adverse outcomes. There was a 48.2% live birth rate in the IVF alone group vs. 50.8% in a group that just received acupuncture on the day of embryo transfer vs. 61.3% in the whole systems TCM group. Biochemical pregnancy rates were also lower in the whole systems TCM group (Hullender Rubin et al. 2015). See the resources section for more of the major studies and their outcomes.

> *When I first started to specialize in fertility in the early 2000s, women (it was mostly women at that time) would come to see fertility acupuncturists only after exhausting the western medical route. And really it should always be the other way around. Try the least invasive techniques like TCM first to optimize your fertility, and this will either lead to pregnancy or have you better prepared should you need western intervention. I now have patients come to see us before they even start trying to get pregnant, which is great because you need to till the soil before you plant the seed.*
> *—Stephanie*

During ART, you will continue with the nutrition and lifestyle suggestions outlined earlier in this book, as well as most of the supplements, unless otherwise advised by your acupuncturist or reproductive endocrinologist. Below we will explain what your acupuncture and herbal schedule will probably look like during various ART treatments.

Acupuncture during ART Cycles

Acupuncture is best started at least three months prior to ART, for both men and women. Oogenesis and spermatogenesis cycles are approximately this long and it's good to begin working with patients at the start of these cycles. Putting the building blocks in place before your IVF schedule is wise, but sometimes not possible. If you don't have a full three months, there is still much that can be done. Below you'll find the basic recommended treatment plans.

Acupuncture for IVF/IUI/timed intercourse.

For women - In vitro fertilization (IVF):
- ❏ Prior to IVF (three months if possible) until stimulation medications begin – weekly
- ❏ During stimulation medications – twice a week
- ❏ Before transfer (0 – 3 days) – one treatment
- ❏ After transfer (0 – 3 days) – one treatment
- ❏ 5 – 7 days after transfer – one treatment
- ❏ Through the first trimester – one treatment every 1 – 2 weeks

---

For women - Timed intercourse/ intrauterine insemination(IUI):
- ❑ Prior to IUI/ovulation (three months if possible) – weekly
- ❑ Before IUI/ovulation (0 – 3 days) – one treatment
- ❑ After IUI/ovulation (0 – 3 days) – one treatment
- ❑ 5 – 7 days after IUI/ovulation – one treatment
- ❑ Through the first trimester – one treatment every 1 – 2 weeks

For men - IVF/IUI/ timed intercourse:
- ❑ Prior to retrieval/IUI/ovulation (three months if possible) – every 1 – 2 weeks
- ❑ 1 – 2 days before ovulation/donation – one treatment

Herbs during ART Cycles

Historically in China, herbal medicine is a very important part of fertility enhancement and treatment, and combining herbs with ART is commonplace there today. It is less common in the western world, although as research continues to show how herbs can raise ART success rates, we are sure to see more fertility clinics allowing their use.

If your acupuncturist feels that it is important for you take herbs at this time, they will talk to your fertility doctor and, if needed, educate them on the use and benefit of Chinese herbs during ART. When this communication occurs, REs are often quite willing to allow their use, especially when it increases their success rates.

Herbs for IVF/IUI/timed intercourse. Taking herbs with IVF or IUI is very dependent on your acupuncturist and your RE, but here are some general guidelines.

For women:
- ❑ You can continue Chinese herbs until you stop the birth control pill. If you do not take the pill, then you can usually take herbs until your suppression check.
- ❑ Discontinue Chinese herbs when you begin stimulation medications (unless otherwise instructed).

❏ Chinese herbal medicine may be prescribed throughout the stimulation medications for various reasons such as past failed cycles.
❏ Once you become pregnant, your herbal prescription will either be discontinued or changed depending on your presenting symptoms.

For men:

❏ Herbs are a very important part of fertility enhancement in Chinese medicine and this is true for men as well. Men can usually be on herbal medicine throughout a woman's fertility cycle.

Supplement and Lifestyle Recommendations during ART Cycles

Discuss the supplement suggestions found in chapter four with your fertility acupuncturist and RE. Once you become pregnant, your acupuncturist will create a new supplement plan for you.

Especially during ART, make sure to keep both your RE and your acupuncturist informed of what you are doing and what you are taking to optimize your fertility. If you have chosen your providers well, they will know what is best for you in regards to your particular diagnosis and situation and may alter your regime.

In the next chapter, we'll discuss how TCM can help with pregnancy and beyond.

9

I'm Pregnant! Now What?

Once you get that positive pregnancy test, Traditional Chinese Medicine (TCM) turns its focus to maintaining the pregnancy and optimizing the overall health of the woman throughout the pregnancy. In this chapter, we will discuss how TCM helps a woman from the first trimester through the postpartum transition and beyond.

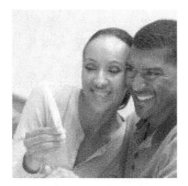

The First Trimester: Securing and Calming the Fetus

"The first trimester can be the most difficult 2 – 3 months of pregnancy, as women often suffer from severe nausea, vomiting, and fatigue. Although these are all signs of a healthy pregnancy, these symptoms can make it difficult to continue on a daily routine. There are medications that can help with nausea, but many women benefit from using acupuncture, acupressure bands, eating ginger or papaya extract and some from chewing gum. Low blood sugar can be a trigger for nausea, and small, frequent meals can help. Also, there is some mind over matter—if something does not look appetizing, it is better to avoid even trying it during the first trimester."—Dr. Judy Kimelman, OB/GYN

In the first trimester, TCM focuses not only on easing symptoms such as nausea, bloating, and fatigue, but on decreasing the risk of miscarriage as well.

The beginning of a pregnancy can be an anxious and stressful time, especially when a couple has struggled to conceive or has had miscarriages in the past. Along with relieving symptoms of pregnancy, acupuncture can help support and calm the anxiety of a newly pregnant woman.

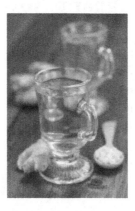

Morning sickness is fairly common in the first trimester, and both herbs and acupuncture can be useful in reducing the nausea and vomiting associated with this early stage of pregnancy. The herbal formulas that are used to reduce morning sickness are safe and have been used for centuries for this purpose.

Arguably the most important goal of TCM in the first trimester is maintaining the pregnancy by reducing the risk of miscarriage. The TCM language for maintaining a pregnancy is "securing and calming the fetus." For patients who have miscarried in the past, this becomes an especially important part of first trimester care.

> *Theresa came to us having lost two prior pregnancies. She experienced the same symptoms with each loss. She began to spot and have cramps around 5 1/2 weeks of pregnancy. She and her husband were taking at least six months to get pregnant each time, so she felt that time was running out. She began fertility enhancement with us, and within two months, she was pregnant again (and nervous). The early weeks went along fine, but when she entered the week of her prior miscarriages, the miscarriage symptoms began. She started to panic and called me. We saw her almost every day for a week. She also took Chinese herbs and did moxibustion (burning of Chinese herbs over certain acupuncture points) at home. After a week, her miscarriage signs went away and she went on to deliver a healthy baby girl. She just returned to the office to start trying for baby number two. —Stephanie*

While TCM works to calm the system and support a pregnancy, it will not prevent the loss of an unhealthy pregnancy (for instance, if the fetus has a genetic issue). If a patient has had miscarriages in the past or is having symptoms that are considered a warning sign in TCM, such as night sweats, then a newly pregnant woman will receive more frequent acupuncture and possibly Chinese herbal medicine to help stabilize the pregnancy.

If the woman starts spotting or bleeding, then the treatment plan is to "calm" the restless fetus and stop the bleeding, as well as send them to see their prenatal care provider.

Fertility acupuncturists treat newly pregnant women with these three goals in mind: reducing anxiety, relieving symptoms such as morning sickness, and decreasing the risk of miscarriage. Frequency of acupuncture treatment during the first trimester depends on several factors, including stage of pregnancy, hormone levels, symptoms, and patient history.

The Second Trimester: The Miraculously Developing Fetus

> *"The second trimester is the 'honeymoon period' of the pregnancy where many women have a resurgence of energy and get the 'glow of pregnancy.' But other women will suffer from headaches throughout the early part of the second trimester. Again, this can be the result of low blood sugar or being dehydrated. Also, some women will develop backaches, sciatica or tension headaches. Massage therapy (or acupuncture) can help alleviate these symptoms. Getting enough sleep is important throughout the rest of the pregnancy since you may feel you are on an emotional roller coaster, and sleep deprivation adds to this feeling. Yoga is a great way to deal with stress, get exercise and add flexibility, which can help in labor. The breathing techniques used in yoga help women later during labor." —Dr. Judy Kimelman, OB/GYN*

The mother usually gets acupuncture at least once a month during her pregnancy to help facilitate the magnificent development of the fetus's physical and energetic self.

The mother is also treated as needed for a variety of ailments that can occur throughout pregnancy, such as back pain, insomnia, pelvic pain, anxiety, constipation, depression, gestational diabetes, hypertension, edema or swelling, GI upset and nausea, headaches, and placenta previa. Acupuncture has been used as an effective treatment for many of the common maladies of pregnancy for thousands of years.

A wonderful tradition of TCM is the "Beautiful Baby Gold Needle Treatment." At the end of both the first and second trimester, TCM offers a traditional acupuncture treatment with gold acupuncture needles to help usher the baby into the next trimester. This treatment focuses on the mother's Kidney energy, which is the wellspring from which babies are nurtured.

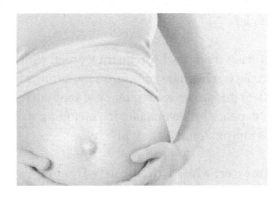

The Third Trimester: Labor Preparation

"Finally you begin the countdown as you enter your third trimester. You are getting close to meeting your baby at last, but often it will feel like your body is betraying you. You will have more difficulty sleeping, walking, and just feeling comfortable as you get bigger. There is a real mixture of emotions as you contemplate labor and delivery and the major changes to your life. Keeping stress as low as possible will help you get through this period of time. Plan to do fewer of the things you would normally do in a week and really use the weekends to catch up on sleep and relaxation." —Dr. Judy Kimelman, OB/GYN

New symptoms can emerge in the third trimester, and TCM can help by relieving the stress, fatigue, and body aches associated with the mother's changing body.

TCM has also been found useful with an issue unique to the third trimester: breech presentation. If your baby is in a breech position, meaning they are not head down, your provider may discuss the option of a C-section for delivery.

TCM, however, has been used successfully to nourish the mother in order to provide an environment where the baby can turn itself from a breech position to a head down position through the use of moxibustion (the process of burning a Chinese herb over specific acupuncture points).

There have been many studies done on the use of moxibustion in creating the environment needed for babies to turn from a breech to a head down position. The most recent study was published in 2013. This study (Vas et al. 2013) showed that in the true moxibustion group, 58.1% of the full-term presentations were head down compared with 43.4% in the sham moxibustion group and 44.8% of those in the usual care group. These studies have been replicated again and again. (See the resources section for a list of those studies).

Preparing for Labor

> *Our patients begin getting acupuncture weekly for labor preparation starting at 35 weeks and twice a week once 40 weeks is reached. —Stephanie*

Once you reach about 35 weeks, it's time to start preparing your body for labor. The goal of TCM in this phase is to get the woman's body as strong as possible to ensure a safe and healthy delivery.

Labor preparation acupuncture involves relaxing muscles and tendons, calming the mind, starting to ripen the cervix, and helping to coax the baby into a head down position. Fertility acupuncturists will also look to TCM in order to see where the woman's imbalances lie and treat those in order to get the woman's body strong for the upcoming labor. For example, if she has swelling, then her spleen is weak and if she is fearful, her kidney energy needs strengthening.

By preparing the mother's body for labor in the month prior to her due date, the goal is for labor to go more smoothly. And it often does—the research backs up these claims. A study done in Austria (Zeisler et al. 1998) showed that acupuncture decreases the actual number of hours a woman spends in labor when acupuncture is performed weekly starting at week 35. The acupuncture group in this study had an average labor time of eight hours, while the control group's average was twelve hours. Acupuncture has also been shown to help ripen the cervix as well as Western medication does (Gribel et al. 2011).

Natural remedies for labor preparation. There are centuries of ideas from various cultures on how to prepare for labor. One of these ideas with at least one study to back it up is that the consumption of dates in the four weeks leading up to delivery can possibly reduce the need for induction (Al-Kuran et al. 2011). And evening primrose oil starting at 34 weeks is thought to help soften the cervix and prepare it for labor as it has prostaglandin-like substances.

Make sure to consult your fertility acupuncturist and prenatal care provider before taking any supplements or medications during pregnancy.

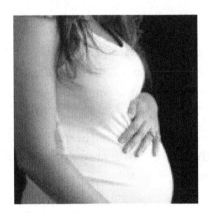

Post-Term Acupuncture

If labor induction is needed, many women opt for natural methods before being medically induced. TCM treatments like acupuncture, herbs, and massage can be used to help induce labor if that is appropriate and supported by your prenatal care provider.

Acupuncture is much more helpful getting labor started when you begin getting treated at least a month prior to your due date. However, in one study where acupuncture started around 39 weeks, the acupuncture group still delivered their babies on average 21 hours sooner than the control group and had an almost 50% reduction in C-sections (Harper et al. 2006).

> **How does sex help induce labor?** Sex is also considered helpful to induce labor although researchers aren't exactly sure why. Some hypotheses include the fact that sperm contains prostaglandins, which are thought to ripen the cervix, and that orgasm and physical stimulation during sex releases oxytocin (Kavanagh et al. 2001). Nipple stimulation or using a breast pump also releases oxytocin, which can reduce stress hormones, as well as stimulate contractions and keep labor going once it starts.

Consult your TCM practitioner and prenatal care provider before actively trying to induce contractions or labor with any technique.

Acupuncture during Labor

Acupuncture during labor is used to minimize pain. One study showed that acupuncture performed during labor was not only appreciated by 87% of the laboring women and well tolerated by 83% of the labor and delivery nurses (who thought that 78% of the women benefited from the acupuncture), but C-section rates dropped by over half (Citkovitz et al. 2009). Not all hospitals allow acupuncture on site, but the number that do is growing. If you are interested in acupuncture during labor, ask your fertility acupuncturist, OB/GYN, midwife or doula for a referral, as it is a specialty in and of itself.

The Fourth Trimester: Postpartum and the Confinement Period

The postpartum period is often called "the fourth trimester" of pregnancy. Your new baby has finally arrived after all this planning and preparation, and it might be more than a little exhausting. Maybe you are having trouble breastfeeding, or you are in pain from an episiotomy or C-section. It may be stressful and overwhelming trying to balance body changes and caring for an infant with disrupted sleep, but TCM care doesn't end when the baby is born. Acupuncturists have a lot to offer the new mother and child, including help with nursing, recovery from delivery, and relief from anxiety and fatigue.

TCM has specific post-natal treatments for both new mother and baby. Besides help with issues that may arise such as pain, lactation problems, depression or exhaustion, TCM invokes its long-standing belief in preventative medicine by advocating for a one-month confinement period for mother and child, as both are vulnerable after childbirth.

TCM considers childbirth to lead to loss of Qi and Blood, so replenishment is needed. The confinement period is meant to accelerate healing post-birth, strengthen the mother, and prevent postpartum health issues. Below are some of the suggestions from Traditional Chinese Medicine given during the confinement period.

Acupuncture

Acupuncture can help with a wide range of postpartum issues, including lactation problems (Wei et al. 2008), mastitis, episiotomy pain (Marra et al. 2011), energy loss, urinary problems, hemorrhoids, depression (Chung et al. 2012) and anxiety, post-delivery pain, and weakened immunity.

If there is an acupuncturist in your area who makes house calls, then acupuncture is recommended as soon as three days post delivery (for women who have had an uncomplicated vaginal birth). Women who have had a C-section usually wait at least a week post delivery to begin getting acupuncture.

Babies can begin receiving TCM care (massage and occasionally herbs instead of acupuncture) within the first month for issues such as colic, ear infections, other digestive issues and trouble sleeping. In metropolitan areas, you should be able to find an acupuncturist who specializes in pediatrics.

Nutrition

Chinese medicine is very engaged in regaining the strength of the new mother. During the confinement period, she is meant to eat warming foods that are easy to digest. Soups and broths (that she does not prepare) are the perfect postpartum foods for the new mother. She should eat balanced meals and snacks and avoid foods that are greasy, fatty, cold or spicy. She is also meant to reduce supplement, herb, caffeine, and alcohol intake. No nicotine is allowed.

Lifestyle

The new mother and child are meant to stay indoors and avoid cold and drafts because the woman is vulnerable after childbirth and it is easy for the cold to get in and further weaken her. She should also avoid heavy exercise and sweating. Indeed, a new mother in the confinement period is meant to do nothing except nourish herself and feed her child. Everything else is done for her.

Although we in the West may find the confinement period to be a bit extreme and even, well, confining, the idea behind it is a good one: protect and strengthen both mother and child after the strenuous ordeal of childbirth.

What recovery will look like for each individual mother and child will be different, but what we can learn from this long-standing tradition is to protect the child as she acclimates to her new surroundings and gains strength to be out in the world and to allow the mother to fully recuperate and protect her future health. TCM at its best is preventative medicine and the postpartum confinement period perfectly illustrates that concept.

Summary

As you can see, Traditional Chinese Medicine helps in all aspects of the fertility, pregnancy, and postpartum journey. Whether you choose an Eastern or Western approach to fertility enhancement or a combination of the two, we wish you a balanced and positive journey towards starting or completing your family!

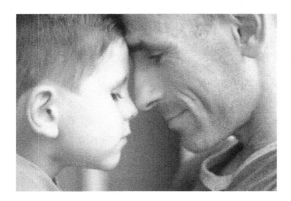

Appendix One

What is Your Chinese Medicine Diagnosis?

This quiz is meant to help you find your Chinese medicine diagnosis. Answer yes or no to each of the following questions. Don't worry about what the symptoms mean; just note whether you experience them. If you have more than one-third yes responses in any diagnostic category, then you may have an element of this imbalance in your system. At the end of each section, you'll find dietary recommendations for each deficiency.

You may have more than one kind of imbalance at the same time, so don't be surprised if you have 50 percent yes answers for more than one diagnostic category. Not all of these categories are discussed in the book, but you can mention your quiz results to your fertility acupuncturist.

KIDNEY YIN DEFICIENCY

- ❑ Do you have lower back weakness, soreness or pain, or knee problems?
- ❑ Do you have ringing in your ears or dizziness?
- ❑ Has your hair gone prematurely gray?
- ❑ Do you have dark circles around or under your eyes?
- ❑ Do you have night sweats?
- ❑ Are you prone to hot flashes?
- ❑ Would you describe yourself as afraid a lot?
- ❑ Does your tongue lack coating? Does it appear shiny or peeled?
- ❑ My skin, hair, and/or nails are dry.
- ❑ My mouth and throat often feel dry.
- ❑ I have dry eyes.
- ❑ I often feel hot.
- ❑ I sometimes feel feverish in the afternoon.
- ❑ I wake up during the night.
- ❑ I am often thirsty.
- ❑ I tend to be constipated.
- ❑ My bowel movements are hard and dry.

- ❏ I prefer colder weather.
- ❏ Given the choice, I would prefer a cold drink.
- ❏ My hands and feet tend to be hot or sweaty.
- ❏ My chest sweats, especially at night.
- ❏ I flush easily or have a red face.
- ❏ I often feel anxious or uneasy; I am a worrywart.
- ❏ I am thin.
- ❏ I am restless and fidgety.
- ❏ I am tired a lot.
- ❏ I am a restless sleeper.
- ❏ I have vivid dreams.

Dietary recommendations for Kidney Yin Deficiency
Yin is the fluid of the body (of which Blood is a part) and it is strengthened by foods like avocados, pears, eggs, mangoes, and pomegranates.

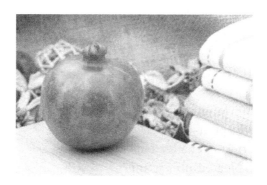

KIDNEY YANG DEFICIENCY

- ❏ Is your low back sore or weak?
- ❏ Are your feet cold, especially at night?
- ❏ Are you typically colder than those around you?
- ❏ Is your libido low?
- ❏ Are you often fearful?
- ❏ Do you wake up at night or early in the morning because you have to urinate?
- ❏ Do you urinate frequently, and is the urine diluted and/or profuse?
- ❏ Do you have early morning, loose, urgent stools?

❑ Do you feel cold cramps during your period that respond to a heating pad?

❑ Is your tongue pale, moist, and swollen?

Dietary recommendations for Kidney Yang Deficiency
Yang is the heat of the body. Foods that build heat include walnuts, shrimp, lamb, garlic and ginger.

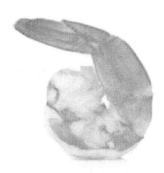

SPLEEN QI DEFICIENCY

❑ Are you often fatigued?

❑ Do you have a poor appetite?

❑ Is your energy lower after a meal?

❑ Do you feel bloated after eating?

❑ Do you crave sweets?

❑ Do you have loose stools, abdominal pain, or digestive problems?

❑ Are your hands and feet cold?

❑ Is your nose cold?

❑ Are you prone to feeling heavy or sluggish?

❑ Are you prone to feeling heaviness or grogginess in the head?

❑ Do you bruise easily?

❑ Do you think you have poor circulation?

❑ Do you have varicose veins?

❑ Are you lacking strength in your arms and legs?

❑ Are you lacking in exercise?

❑ Are you prone to worry?

❑ Have you been diagnosed with low blood pressure?

❑ Do you sweat a lot without exerting yourself?

- ❑ Do you feel dizzy or lightheaded, or have visual changes when you stand up fast?
- ❑ Are you often sick, or do you have allergies?
- ❑ Have you been diagnosed with hypothyroid or anemia?
- ❑ Do you have hemorrhoids or polyps?
- ❑ Does your tongue look swollen, with teeth marks on the sides?
- ❑ Do you have a pale, yellowish complexion?

Dietary recommendations for Spleen Qi Deficiency
Foods that tonify Qi include dates, squash, oats, and sweet potato.

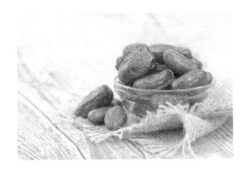

BLOOD DEFICIENCY (not necessarily equated with anemia)

- ❑ Do you have dry, flaky skin?
- ❑ Are you prone to getting chapped lips?
- ❑ Are you losing hair on your head (not in patches, but all over)?
- ❑ Is your hair brittle or dry?
- ❑ Do you have diminished nighttime vision?
- ❑ Are your lips, the inner side of your lower eyelids, or tongue pale in color?
- ❑ My nail beds are pale, and my nails are dry and break easily.
- ❑ I get dizzy easily, especially if I stand up quickly.
- ❑ I have blurry vision or floaters.
- ❑ I have trouble falling asleep.
- ❑ I am tired.
- ❑ My hair is thin and/or dry.
- ❑ I am a vegan or vegetarian.
- ❑ Sometimes I get palpitations.

- ❏ I often feel shaky.
- ❏ My muscles are tight, and it doesn't take much for me to injure them.

Dietary recommendations for Blood Deficiency
Red foods tonify Blood in TCM, so think organ meats, beets, red chard, and dark berries.

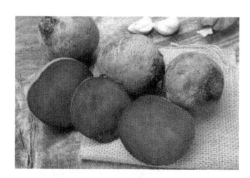

LIVER QI STAGNATION

- ❏ Are you prone to emotional depression?
- ❏ Are you prone to anger and/or rage?
- ❏ Are your pupils usually dilated and large?
- ❏ Do you have difficulty falling asleep at night?
- ❏ Do you experience heartburn or wake up with a bitter taste in your mouth?
- ❏ Is your tongue dark or purplish in color?
- ❏ I am often irritable.
- ❏ I feel tense, overwhelmed, or just generally stuck.
- ❏ My bowel movements are thin and long like a ribbon.
- ❏ My bowel movements are like small pebbles.
- ❏ My ribs or flanks are painful or distended.
- ❏ I feel better or have more energy with exercise.
- ❏ I am stressed out.
- ❏ I sigh a lot.
- ❏ I grind my teeth at night.
- ❏ I have tense muscles.
- ❏ I have poor circulation.
- ❏ I feel as if I can't quite clear my throat.

- ❏ I have a nervous stomach and feel nauseous or get diarrhea when I'm stressed.
- ❏ I have cold hands and feet.

Dietary recommendations for Liver Qi Stagnation

Most people have some Liver Qi Stagnation, but if you have an extreme case of it, it is more important to avoid certain foods rather than adding foods. Foods and drinks to avoid include alcohol, greasy food, and spicy food. These foods may give you temporary relief, but will further stagnate the Liver in the long run.

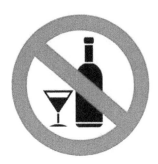

HEART DEFICIENCY (often associated with heat)

- ❏ Do you wake up early in the morning and have trouble getting back to sleep?
- ❏ Do you have heart palpitations, especially when anxious?
- ❏ Do you have nightmares?
- ❏ Do you seem low in spirit or lacking in vitality?
- ❏ Are you prone to agitation or extreme restlessness?
- ❏ Do you fidget?
- ❏ Is the tip of your tongue red?
- ❏ Is there a crack in the center of your tongue that extends to the tip?
- ❏ Do you sweat excessively, especially on your chest?

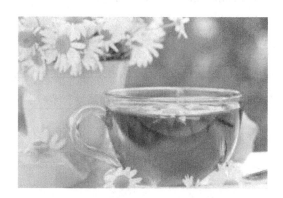

EXCESS HEAT

- ❏ Is your pulse rate rapid?
- ❏ Are your mouth and throat usually dry?
- ❏ Are you thirsty for cold drinks most of the time?
- ❏ Do you often feel warmer than those around you?
- ❏ Do you wake up sweating or have hot flashes?
- ❏ Do you break out with red acne?

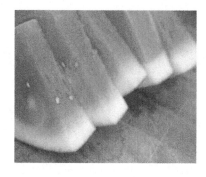

DAMPNESS

- ❏ Do you feel tired and sluggish after a meal?
- ❏ Do you have cystic or pustular acne?
- ❏ Do you have urgent, bright, or foul-smelling stools?
- ❏ Do your joints ache, especially with movement?
- ❏ Are you overweight?
- ❏ Do you have a wet, slimy tongue?
- ❏ I have trouble controlling my weight.
- ❏ My thinking often feels clouded.
- ❏ I have sinus problems, seasonal allergies, or a chronic cough.
- ❏ I have a tendency toward edema, or swelling.
- ❏ My hands or feet swell.
- ❏ I often feel tired and sluggish.
- ❏ I get achy joints.
- ❏ My arms and legs feel heavy.
- ❏ My urine is cloudy.
- ❏ I feel bloated.

Dietary recommendations for Dampness
Foods that drain dampness include radishes, celery, mushrooms, and aduki beans. Make sure that you are reducing intake of damp-producing foods such as soy and dairy.

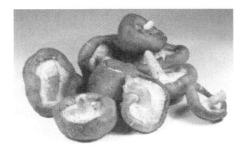

Appendix Two

TCM Dietary Guidelines

Traditional Chinese medical doctors have long recognized the importance of diet and digestion in maintaining health and preventing disease (please note that these guidelines are not meant to substitute for dietary guidelines given by your doctor for a health condition such as diabetes or renal disease). Here are a few time-tested pearls of wisdom.

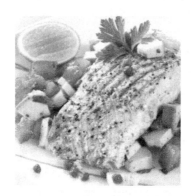

- ❏ **Food and drinks that are cold in temperature injure the digestive process**. Your digestive system is like a cooking pot. Adding icy drinks, ice cream, and smoothies to this "pot" slows down your digestion and requires more energy for your body to warm up and "cook" your food. Room temperature drinks are recommended. Spicy flavors such as pepper, ginger, and cinnamon can counteract "cold" food and drinks.
- ❏ **Salads, most raw fruits, and raw vegetables are difficult for the body to digest**. They require more energy from your digestive system to break down. By steaming and/or cooking vegetables and eating raw fruit in moderation, your body has better access to the nutrition in food.
- ❏ **Eat on a regular schedule**. Your body's enzymes and hormones are secreted at certain times of the day. Eating at a regular time can help your body prepare for digesting and breaking down food you eat.

Late-night eating wreaks havoc on your digestive system (and can lead to a restless night of sleep).

❏ **Eat until you're satiated, but not overly full.** Overloading your stomach with food can overwhelm your digestive system. If there is a little extra room inside, your stomach can more easily break down your food.

❏ **Too much milk, sugar, wheat, and greasy, fried, or spicy foods can contribute to sluggishness and chronic health complaints.** These foods can contribute to mucus production, excess fluids, growth of bacteria, pain in the joints, fatigue, heaviness, and inflammation. Sugar is abundant in many foods and can be addictive. Eliminating some or all of these foods can cause a dramatic increase in energy and vitality.

❏ **A balance of flavors keeps the body in balance (and makes food delicious).** Too much of any one taste (sweet, salty, sour, spicy, astringent) can cause an imbalance internally. Ideally, meals should have a nice balance of all of these flavors. For example: a tuna salad with lemon juice (sour), celery and pepper (spicy), apple slices (sweet), and a touch of vinegar (astringent).

❏ **Eat according to your TCM diagnosis.** Once you have a TCM diagnosis, you can begin to add foods to your diet that will strengthen and balance your body.

This appendix was written by Cheryl House, LAc, FABORM of Acupuncture Northwest & Associates in Seattle, Washington.

Appendix Three

Understanding Your Digestion Through The Middle Burner

What is the Middle Burner? A Chinese medicine look at your digestive system

In Chinese Medicine, the middle burner is the heart of the digestive system. A vivid image of the middle burner is a wood-burning stove that heats a house. Digestion is the stove, and food is the fuel. The quality of the fuel determines the efficiency of the stove and therefore the warmth of the house, i.e. the health and energy of the body.

Is there a Western equivalent?

The equivalent to an efficient middle-burner in Western medicine is an effective metabolism. Good metabolism will "burn" the food cleanly, utilizing calories, burning fat, and assimilating vitamins and nutrients, giving the body energy for living. If your metabolism is appropriate for your activities and food intake, you will naturally maintain your optimal weight.

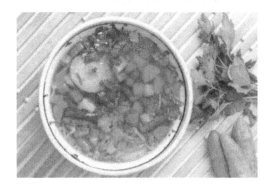

What benefits the digestive fire?

When you wake up in the morning, the fire in your stove has reduced to embers. The fire must be stoked to carry out its digestive function.

Breakfast: To build a strong fire, the day begins with breakfast, which acts as kindling. In Chinese medicine, hot, whole grain cereal, congee, is an ideal meal to gently start your digestive metabolism for clean, efficient, warm burning.

Lunch: The digestive fire is the strongest at lunchtime. Lunch should therefore be the biggest meal of the day, with the most variety. It should contain concentrated protein such as animal products, legumes, nuts, and seeds.

Dinner: The last meal should ideally be the smallest. It's best if the meal is eaten before 7pm, and that the meal is cooked. A good example is steamed vegetables and a grain.

What injures the middle burner?
- ❏ A large, heavy breakfast is like throwing a big oak log on a struggling, flickering flame; it might be snuffed.
- ❏ Cold cereal and milk is like throwing wet, soggy leaves on a tender little fire.
- ❏ Fried eggs and hash browns is like green wood; it burns poorly and produces thick, noxious smoke.
- ❏ Not eating breakfast would certainly put the fire out for the day as it needs fuel to burn.
- ❏ Ice-cold drinks and foods like ice cream also destroy the digestive fire.

If you tend to your middle burner as if you were tending a fire, you will be able to achieve and maintain your health and ideal body weight.

Appendix Four

The Issue of Pesticides and Chinese Herbal Medicine

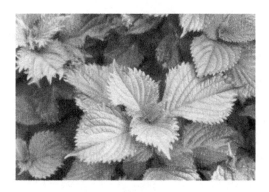

Many patients, especially when they are pregnant, are rightly concerned about environmental toxins that could potentially contaminate the Chinese herbs they are being given. While this does warrant consideration, please note that all Chinese herbs that come into the United States are tested for pesticides and most test lower than non-organic fruit and vegetables. It's a complicated issue, with some herbs faring better than others.

At Acupuncture Northwest, we mainly use whole herbs and get organic when possible. We then tincture them so we know what the herb looked like before we processed it into a Western patient-friendly version. We occasionally send for the import document from the herb company that shows the levels of different chemicals found on the herbs. And again, normally these levels are less than a non-organic vegetable.

> **Research on the safety of Chinese herbal medicine.** In a 2011 study of Chinese Herbal Medicine, 95% of the herbs tested were considered safe according to standard TCM dosing (Harris et al. 2011). In an article in *Acupuncture Today*, a newspaper for TCM practitioners, the author noted that you are more likely to have a long-term effect from the fruits and

vegetables you eat over the course of your life than from the Chinese herbs
that you consume on a shorter-term basis (Brand 2014).

At Acupuncture Northwest, we mainly use the KPC brand for our powdered
herbs, which is a company that operates out of Taiwan. You can find their
testing protocols on their website at www.craneherb.com. For our raw herbs
that we tincture, we feel confident that Andrew Ellis' company, Spring Wind,
is getting us the cleanest herbs that it can. You can find their testing protocols
at springwind.com/quality-control. We occasionally request testing reports
from both of these companies. We use the Golden Flower company out of
New Mexico for any herbal formulas in pill form. Their testing for microbes,
pesticide residue, heavy metals and potency can be found on their website at
gfcherbs.com.

We have carefully chosen these brands, and we feel confident in using them.
We also believe that the way plants, both food and herbs alike, are grown on
this planet would be better if we moved towards more ecological farming.

Bottom line? Find a fertility acupuncturist that you trust and make sure they
are getting their herbs from a reputable source.

Appendix Five

Finding Your Fertility Care Providers

Finding a Good Fertility Acupuncturist

If you want to start adding Traditional Chinese Medicine to your journey to start a family, the first step is finding the right fertility acupuncturist. You want an experienced, compassionate fertility acupuncturist, someone who is focused on women's health as well as fertility for both men and women.

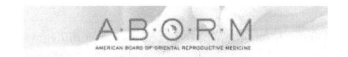

Your fertility acupuncturist should be board certified with the American Board of Oriental Reproductive Medicine (ABORM). Not all great fertility acupuncturists have this credential, but it does ensure that your acupuncturist is specialized in the area of fertility enhancement.

ABORM certified acupuncturists have spent extensive time learning about the treatment of infertility with TCM and have passed a national exam. They must do continuing education to keep their ABORM credential current. You can find an ABORM certified practitioner by going to the ABORM website at www.aborm.org and looking under your location. There are ABORM credentialed practitioners in the United States, Canada, Australia, and Europe.

Because fertility enhancement often involves collaboration with Western physicians, it is best to find a fertility acupuncturist who has a good relationship with the best Western medicine fertility clinics in your area. You should be able to find this out by looking at either the acupuncturist's or the fertility clinic's website. If you are going to a fertility clinic, you can also ask your specialist there for a recommendation.

Experience is key. Fertility enhancement acupuncture and the treatment of infertility with Chinese medicine is a very specialized field with change occurring rapidly in both Western medicine and Western alternative medicine. You will need an acupuncturist who focuses on reproductive medicine and TCM but who also keeps abreast of the latest research in the Western realm. Your fertility acupuncturist needs to know how to read your fertility focused lab values (such as AMH, FSH and estradiol) and help guide you through the sometimes confusing world of ART.

So start by asking for referrals and then do your own research to see which of your referrals also has the above qualifications. Once you find the right fertility acupuncturist, you will be glad that you did!

Finding a Good Fertility Doctor (Reproductive Endocrinologist)

Finding the right fertility doctor is an important step in your fertility journey. That person should not only have the appropriate training and expertise in the field of fertility but also provide compassionate care.

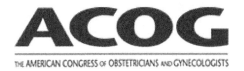

Some primary care providers, including midwives and obstetricians, will have some experience with fertility and may be able to help you get started with an evaluation. You should be aware that many providers have not been trained in fertility or they have not kept up to date on the latest testing and treatment options available.

Be direct when you are asking for help with fertility and ask your provider how much experience they have had with fertility patients. Make sure they feel comfortable getting the right tests and making the right treatment plans for you—a good provider will know their limitations and refer you to a different provider when appropriate.

A Western medicine fertility expert is called a reproductive endocrinologist. A reproductive endocrinologist is someone with specialized training, including four years in medical school, a four year residency training in Obstetrics and Gynecology, and a subsequent three year fellowship in Reproductive Endocrinology and Infertility. Less than 50 reproductive endocrinologists complete fellowship training each year in the United States.

Beyond training, Western medical doctors are expected to become board certified in their specialized area of medicine. A reproductive endocrinologist has the opportunity to be double board certified, meaning they are not only board certified in the field of Obstetrics and Gynecology but also board certified in the field of Reproductive Endocrinology and Infertility.

Board certification is a rigorous process involving two intense evaluations: a written exam followed by an oral exam in which experts in the field ask the candidate questions about the field but also require the candidate to defend their research in the field. The board certification process can take several years to complete. Some providers may be 'board eligible,' which means they have finished their training and are capable of providing good care, but they have not yet completed all the steps of being board certified.

With all this training and experience, most reproductive endocrinologists have the knowledge to provide good fertility care. Finding the right reproductive endocrinologist for you will mean doing some research and investigation. Ask your fertility acupuncturist or your primary care provider for recommendations. Ask your friends and read online. Make sure you use several sources. You should be able to find someone with not only the academic training, but the ability to provide compassionate care.

Glossary of Terms and Acronyms

Acupuncture: A Traditional Chinese Medicine (TCM) treatment that involves using hair-thin needles inserted at key points along Qi pathways to encourage energy and blood flow throughout the body.

Anti-Müllerian hormone (AMH): A hormone found in the ovaries that may tested as part of the Western fertility treatment process. In general, AMH is considered a quantitative assessment of ovarian reserve. A low AMH is associated with a lower response to ovarian stimulation medication. AMH is a relatively new ovarian reserve test and interpretation is still under investigation.

Antioxidants: Molecules that decrease oxidative stress in the body, such as vitamin C, vitamin E, alpha lipoic acid, N-acetylcysteine, and melatonin.

Antral Follicle Count: The number of follicles that can be seen in both ovaries with the use of a transvaginal ultrasound. A low antral follicle count may indicate a low ovarian reserve and a diminished response to ovarian stimulation medication.

Aneuploid: A term used to describe an incorrect match of chromosomes within an embryo. Each embryo should have two copies of each chromosome—one from the egg and one from the sperm.

Assisted Reproductive Technology (ART): Methods of conceiving with artificial or partially artificial means. ART options essentially involve ovarian stimulation with medication followed by intrauterine insemination (IUI) or in vitro fertilization (IVF). ART is used by western medicine practitioners as the primary means for helping a couple conceive.

ATP (adenosine triphosphate): The energy for many processes within all the cells in our body. The process of egg maturation, DNA replication, fertilization and all cellular processes require ATP.

Basal Body Temperature (BBT): A means of tracking temperature fluctuations throughout the month by taking a woman's temperature every morning at the same time in order to track ovulation and assess the lengths of both the follicular and the luteal phase. Your acupuncturist will also use these temperatures for TCM diagnostic purposes.

Blastocyst: The embryo stage on day 5-6 after ovulation.

Cervical Factor Infertility: Infertility due to a cervix that filters too well due to decreased secretions or scar tissue.

Chromosome: The part of the cell that carries your DNA.

Cofactor: Helper molecules that help in biochemical transformations.

Cryopreservation: The process of freezing eggs, sperm, or embryos for future use (sometimes used with the IVF procedure).

Cycle Day (CD): A way of tracking where you are in your cycle. Cycle day 1 begins on the first day of full flow and is signalled by a temperature drop, if you are taking your temperature every morning (see BBT).

Diminished Ovarian Reserve (DOR): Ovarian reserve is the ability of the ovaries to provide healthy, viable eggs which have the capacity to fertilize and result in healthy, successful pregnancies. Diminished ovarian reserve is essentially a lower number of eggs or follicles and a lower than expected response to ovarian stimulation medication for a woman than predicted by age alone. No universal definition of diminished ovarian reserve has been agreed upon, but elevated FSH levels and low AMH levels and antral follicles counts are associated with poor response to ovarian stimulation treatment and thus diminished ovarian reserve.

Essence: A Traditional Chinese Medicine term used to describe your Kidney energy, which can also be thought of as your bank account of Qi out of which babies are made, for both men and women.

Follicle Stimulating Hormone (FSH): A hormone that promotes the formation of eggs and sperm. FSH is a fairly good predictor of ovarian reserve in women, and should be tested early in the cycle, usually cycle day three (the third day of menstrual bleeding). A high FSH is associated with diminished ovarian reserve. Estradiol should be checked with the FSH to ensure accuracy. A high estradiol level can falsely lower a FSH level and mask diminished ovarian reserve.

Follicular Phase: The time from the onset of menses until ovulation.

Four Pillars of Treatment: The four pillars is a term that is used in many different ways within TCM. Within this text, however, the four pillars of TCM treatment include acupuncture, herbal medicine, nutritional advice, and lifestyle suggestions.

Gonadotropin Medications: Injectable medications given in the beginning of the cycle to recruit multiple eggs. Unlike the oral medications that 'trick' the body into producing more follicle-stimulating hormone (FSH), the gonadotropins actually are FSH.

Granulosa cells: Cells that are found in the ovaries that are the supporting cells of developing eggs and also produce AMH.

Hysterosalpingogram (HSG): A test used by ART practitioners that can show the inner shape of the uterus and whether the fallopian tubes are open or not.

Infertility: Infertility is defined as the inability to conceive after 12 months of trying.

Intracytoplasmic Sperm Injection (ICSI): An active method of fertilizing, in which one sperm is injected into one mature egg by an embryologist, sometimes used during the IVF procedure.

Intrauterine Insemination (IUI): IUI is an ART procedure that involves washing/preparing the sperm and placing it with a catheter past the cervix into the uterine cavity during ovulation to increase chances of conception.

In Vitro Fertilization (IVF): The process of conception that involves retrieving eggs out of the body, creating embryos in the IVF lab, and then replacing the embryo(s) into the uterine cavity for implantation.

Luteal Phase: The phase of a woman's cycle from ovulation to the onset of menses.

Luteal Phase Defect (LPD): The luteal phase should ideally last 12 – 14 days. If the luteal phase is shorter than this, it is called a luteal phase defect.

Luteinizing Hormone (LH): A hormone released from the pituitary gland to signal the final maturation and release or ovulation of the egg, important in timing conception.

Meridians: In Traditional Chinese Medicine, meridians are pathways along which your life energy or Qi flows.

Moxibustion: A Traditional Chinese Medicine treatment that involves burning Chinese herbs over certain acupuncture points to stimulate, strengthen and warm particular acupuncture points in order to bring the body more towards health.

Oogenesis: The formation and maturation of the ovum (egg).

Organ Systems: In Traditional Chinese Medicine, the organ systems are a complex of structures and energy that work together and include both the actual organ as well as the corresponding meridian.

Ovarian Hyperstimulation Syndrome (OHSS): A condition that can occur as a side effect among women who take ovarian stimulation medications during ART treatments. OHSS can cause the ovaries to become swollen and painful, and a small number of women may experience more severe symptoms such as vomiting, abdominal pain, or shortness of breath.

Ovarian Reserve: The ability of the ovaries to provide healthy, viable eggs which have the capacity to fertilize and result in healthy, successful pregnancies.

Ovulation Induction: Ovulation induction involves giving medication in the early follicular phase (starting within the first 2 – 5 days of menses) in order to recruit more than one egg to ovulate.

Ovulation Predictor Kits (OPKs): Also called fertility monitors, OPKs turn positive when the pituitary gland releases a surge of luteinizing hormone, signalling ovulation.

Polycystic Ovary Syndrome (PCOS): PCOS is a common hormonal disorder among women. Although not all women with PCOS experience the same symptoms, some of the common symptoms include infertility, missing or irregular periods, chronic high testosterone (often indicated by excess facial and body hair, acne, and hair loss on the scalp), and small cysts in the ovaries that contain immature eggs.

Preimplantation Genetic Diagnosis: Genetic testing of embryos for specific diseases, which can be used in conjunction with IVF.

Premature Ovarian Failure (POF): The loss of normal ovarian function before the age of 40, often resulting in menopause-like symptoms, irregular or missing periods, and infertility issues.

Qi: Vital energy or life force, pronounced "chee." Within TCM and indeed in China, everything nonliving or living is infused with Qi. Qi permeates the universe. In the West, Qi often refers to the energy that imbues living things that cannot be seen but we know are there. Qi courses through the body's meridians, makes the heart beat and gives life to the spirit and body.

Recurrent Pregnancy Loss (RPL): The ASRM defines recurrent pregnancy loss as two or more clinical pregnancy losses before the pregnancy reaches 20 weeks.

Reproductive Endocrinologist (RE): An OB/GYN who has undergone additional training in order to diagnose and treat infertility issues. REs have completed medical school, a residency training in the field of obstetrics and gynecology, and subsequent sub-specialty training in the form of a fellowship in reproductive endocrinology and infertility.

Sperm Parameters: These include sperm count, motility (their ability to move), morphology (their shape) and other parameters that are helpful in determining male fertility.

Spermatogenesis: The formation and maturation of sperm.

Traditional Chinese Medicine (TCM): An ancient medicine based on at least 3000 years of experience that uses poetic metaphors to describe human vitality and illness. TCM treatment to regain health, preserve wellness or prevent disease includes the four pillars of treatment: acupuncture, herbal medicine, nutritional advice (food as medicine) and lifestyle suggestions.

Transvaginal Ultrasound: An ultrasound that is used to look at and evaluate a woman's reproductive organs.

Varicocele: An enlargement of the veins within the scrotum that can cause decreased sperm production and quality.

Vitrification: A fast-freezing method of cryopreservation that, if done by highly skilled embryologists, results in very high embryo survival rates (97% or higher) and similar or higher pregnancy rates than the rates for fresh embryo transfer.

Research, Sources and Additional Information

Recommendations for Further Reading

- ❏ *It Starts with the Egg* by Rebecca Fett
- ❏ *The Infertility Cure* by Randine Lewis, LAc
- ❏ *Making Babies* by Jill Blakeway, LAc, and Sami David, MD
- ❏ *The Tao of Fertility* by Daoshing Ni, LAc
- ❏ *Taking Charge of Your Fertility* by Toni Weschler, MPH

Acupuncture and Chinese Herbal Medicine Fertility Research

1. Blood Flow to the Uterus and Acupuncture Research
2. Breech Research
3. Chinese Herbal Medicine and Fertility Research
4. Female Fertility Research
5. IVF and Acupuncture Research
6. Labor Preparation Research
7. Lactation and Acupuncture Research
8. Male Factor Infertility Research
9. PCOS and Acupuncture Research
10. Postpartum Depression and Acupuncture Research
11. Pregnancy and Acupuncture Research

1. Blood Flow to the Uterus and Acupuncture Research

Stener-Victorin E, Waldenström U, Andersson SA, Wikland M. 1996. Reduction of blood flow impedance in the uterine arteries of infertile women with electro-acupuncture. *Hum Reprod.* 11(6):1314-7.
CONCLUSION(S): Compared to the mean baseline PI (pulsatility index), the mean PI was significantly reduced both shortly after the eighth EA treatment (P < 0.0001) and 10-14 days after the EA period (P < 0.0001).

2. Breech Research

Cardini F, Weixin H. 1998. Moxibustion for correction of breech presentation: a randomized controlled trial. *JAMA.* 280(18):1580-4.

CONCLUSION(S): Among primigravidas with breech presentation during the 33rd week of gestation, moxibustion for 1 to 2 weeks increased fetal activity during the treatment period and cephalic presentation after the treatment period and at delivery.

Habek D, Cerkez Habek J, and Jagust M. 2003. Acupuncture conversion of fetal breech presentation. *Fetal Diagn Ther.* 18(6):418-21.
CONCLUSION(S): We believe that AP correction of fetal malpresentation is a relatively simple, efficacious and inexpensive method associated with a lower percentage of operatively completed deliveries, which definitely reflects in improved parameters of vital and perinatal statistics.

Neri I, Airola G, Contu G, Allais G, Facchinetti F, Benedetto C. 2004. Acupuncture plus moxibustion to resolve breech presentation: a randomized controlled study. *J Matern Fetal Neonatal Med.* 15(4):247-52.
CONCLUSION(S): Acupuncture plus moxibustion is more effective than observation in revolving fetuses in breech presentation. Such a method appears to be a valid option for women willing to experience a natural birth.

Vas J, Aranda-Regules JM, Modesto M, Ramos-Monserrat M, Barón M, Aguilar I, Benítez-Parejo N, Ramírez-Carmona C, Rivas-Ruiz F. 2013. Using moxibustion in primary healthcare to correct non-vertex presentation: a multicentre randomised controlled trial. *Acupunct Med.* 31(1):31-8.
CONCLUSION(S): Moxibustion at acupuncture point BL67 is effective and safe to correct non-vertex presentation when used between 33 and 35 weeks of gestation. We believe that moxibustion represents a treatment option that should be considered to achieve version of the non-vertex fetus.

3. Chinese Herbal Medicine Fertility Research

Ried K, Stuart K. 2011. Efficacy of Traditional Chinese Herbal Medicine in the management of female infertility: a systematic review. *Complement Ther Med.* 19(6):319-31.
CONCLUSION(S): Our review suggests that management of female infertility with Chinese Herbal Medicine can improve pregnancy rates two-fold within a four month period compared with Western Medical fertility drug therapy or IVF. Assessment of the quality of the menstrual cycle, integral to TCM diagnosis, appears to be fundamental to successful treatment of female infertility.

See CJ, McCulloch M, Smikle C, Gao J. 2011. Chinese herbal medicine and clomiphene citrate for anovulation: a meta-analysis of randomized controlled trials. *J Altern Complement Med.* 17(5):397-405.
CONCLUSION(S): Chinese herbal medicine may increase the effectiveness of CC therapy. However, the RCTs are of poor methodological quality and small sample size, and the results require confirmation with rigorously controlled studies.

4. Female Fertility Research

Gui J, Xiong F, Yang W, Li J, Huang G. 2012. Effects of acupuncture on LIF and
IL-12 in rats of implantation failure. *Am J Reprod Immunol.* 67(5):383-90.
CONCLUSION(S): Acupuncture could improve the poor receptive state of endometrium
by promoting LIF and IL-12 secretion to improve blastocyst implantation.

Ried K, Stuart K. 2011. Efficacy of Traditional Chinese Herbal Medicine in the
management of female infertility: a systematic review. *Complement Ther Med.*
19(6):319-31.
CONCLUSION(S): Our review suggests that management of female infertility with
Chinese Herbal Medicine can improve pregnancy rates two-fold within a four month
period compared with Western Medical fertility drug therapy or IVF. Assessment of the
quality of the menstrual cycle, integral to TCM diagnosis, appears to be fundamental to
successful treatment of female infertility.

Stener-Victorin E, Wu X. 2010. Effects and mechanisms of acupuncture in the
reproductive system. *Auton Neurosci.* 157(1-2):46-51.
ABSTRACT: The use of acupuncture to treat reproductive dysfunction has not been well
investigated. Only a few clinical studies have been reported, most of which are flawed by
poor design and a lack of valid outcome measures and diagnostic criteria, making the
results difficult to interpret. Experimental studies, however, show that acupuncture has
substantial effects on reproductive function. Here we review the possible mechanisms of
action of acupuncture on the reproductive system and its effects on reproductive
dysfunction, focusing in particular on polycystic ovary syndrome, the most common
endocrine and metabolic disorder in women. Clinical and experimental evidence
demonstrates that acupuncture is a suitable alternative or complement to
pharmacological induction of ovulation, without adverse side effects. Clearly,
acupuncture modulates endogenous regulatory systems, including the sympathetic
nervous system, the endocrine system, and the neuroendocrine system. Randomized
clinical trials are warranted to further evaluate the clinical effects of acupuncture in
reproductive disorders.

5. IVF and Acupuncture Research

di Villahermosa DI, Santos LG, Nogueira MB, Vilarino FL, Barbosa CP. 2013.
Influence of acupuncture on the outcomes of in vitro fertilisation when embryo
implantation has failed: a prospective randomised controlled clinical trial. *Acupunct Med.*
31(2):157-61.
RESULTS: The clinical pregnancy rate in the acupuncture group was significantly higher
than that in the control and sham groups (35.7% vs 7.1% vs 10.7%; p=0.0169).
CONCLUSION(S): In this study, acupuncture and moxibustion increased pregnancy
rates when used as an adjuvant treatment in women undergoing IVF, when embryo
implantation had failed.

Hullender Rubin LE, Opsahl MS, Wiemer KE, Mist SD, Caughey AB. 2015.
Impact of whole systems traditional Chinese medicine on in vitro fertilization outcomes.
Reprod Biomed Online. 30(6):602-12.
RESULTS: Live birth rates were 48.2% IVF alone vs. 50.8% acupuncture only vs. 61.3%
whole systems TCM.
ABSTRACT: Patients undergoing IVF may receive either acupuncture or whole-systems
traditional Chinese medicine (WS-TCM) as an adjuvant IVF treatment. WS-TCM is a
complex intervention that can include acupuncture, Chinese herbal medicine, dietary,
lifestyle recommendations. In this retrospective cohort study, 1231 IVF patient records
were reviewed to assess the effect of adjuvant WS-TCM on IVF outcomes compared
among three groups: IVF with no additional treatment; IVF and elective acupuncture on
day of embryo transfer; or IVF and elective WS-TCM. Overall, IVF with adjuvant
WS-TCM was associated with greater odds of live birth in donor and non-donor cycles
(48.2% IVF alone vs. 50.8% acupuncture only vs. 61.3% whole systems TCM).

Magarelli PC, Cridennda DK, Cohen M. 2009. Changes in serum cortisol and
prolactin associated with acupuncture during controlled ovarian hyperstimulation in
women undergoing in vitro fertilization-embryo transfer treatment. Fertil Steril.
92(6):1870-9.
CONCLUSION(S): In this study, there appears to be a beneficial regulation of CORT and
PRL in the Ac group during the medication phase of the IVF treatment with a trend
toward more normal fertile cycle dynamics.

Manheimer E, Zhang G, Udoff L, Haramati A, Langenberg P, Berman BM, Bouter LM.
2008. Effects of acupuncture on rates of pregnancy and live birth among women
undergoing in vitro fertilisation: systematic review and meta-analysis. *BMJ.*
336(7643):545-9.
CONCLUSION(S): Current preliminary evidence suggests that acupuncture given with
embryo transfer improves rates of pregnancy and live birth among women undergoing in
vitro fertilisation.

Paulus WE, Zhang M, Strehler E, El-Danasouri I, Sterzik K. 2002. Influence of
acupuncture on the pregnancy rate in patients who undergo assisted reproduction
therapy. *Fertil Steril.* 77(4):721-4.
CONCLUSION(S): Acupuncture seems to be a useful tool for improving pregnancy rate
after ART.

Stener-Victorin E, Humaidan P. 2006. Use of acupuncture in female infertility and a
summary of recent acupuncture studies related to embryo transfer. *Acupunct Med.*
24(4):157-63.
ABSTRACT: During the last five years, the use of acupuncture in female infertility as an
adjuvant to conventional treatment in assisted reproductive technology (ART) has
increased in popularity. The present paper briefly discusses clinical and experimental data
on the effect of acupuncture on uterine and ovarian blood flow, as an analgesic method
during ART, and on endocrine and metabolic disturbances such as polycystic ovary
syndrome (PCOS). Further it gives a summary of recent studies evaluating the effect of

acupuncture before and after embryo transfer on pregnancy outcome. Of the four published RCTs, three reveal significantly higher pregnancy rates in the acupuncture groups compared with the control groups. But the use of different study protocols makes it difficult to draw definitive conclusions. It seems, however, that acupuncture has a positive effect and no adverse effects on pregnancy outcome.

Westergaard LG, Mao Q, Krogslund M, Sandrini S, Lenz S, Grinsted J. 2006. Acupuncture on the day of embryo transfer significantly improves the reproductive outcome in infertile women: a prospective, randomized trial. *Fertil Steril.* 85(5):1341-6. CONCLUSION(S): Acupuncture on the day of ET significantly improves the reproductive outcome of IVF/ICSI, compared with no acupuncture. Repeating acupuncture on ET day +2 provided no additional beneficial effect.

6. Labor Preparation Research

Gribel GP, Coca-Velarde LG, Moreira de Sá RA. 2011. Electroacupuncture for cervical ripening prior to labor induction: a randomized clinical trial. *Arch Gynecol Obstet.* 283(6):1233-8.
CONCLUSION(S): Our results showed that electroacupuncture can be used to obtain cervical ripening, with similar results as compared with misoprostol, with a significantly higher frequency of vaginal deliveries and without occurrence of obstetric complications.

Harper TC, Coeytaux RR, Chen W, Campbell K, Kaufman JS, Moise KJ, Thorp JM. 2006. A randomized controlled trial of acupuncture for initiation of labor in nulliparous women. *J Matern Fetal Neonatal Med.* 19(8):465-70.
OBJECTIVE: To evaluate the utility of outpatient acupuncture for labor stimulation. RESULTS: Fifty-six women were randomized and completed the study procedures. Race, age, gestational age, and cervical Bishop score were similar in both groups. Mean time to delivery occurred 21 hours sooner in the acupuncture group, but this difference did not reach statistical significance ($p = 0.36$). Compared to controls, women in the acupuncture group tended to be more likely to labor spontaneously (70% vs. 50%, $p = 0.12$) and less likely to deliver by cesarean section (39% vs. 17%, $p = 0.07$). Of women who were not induced, those in the acupuncture group were more likely to be delivered than the controls at any point after enrollment ($p = 0.05$).
CONCLUSION(S): Acupuncture is well tolerated among term nulliparous women and holds promise in reducing interventions that occur in post-term pregnancies.

Rabl M, Ahner R, Bitschnau M, Zeisler H, Husslein P. 2001. Acupuncture for cervical ripening and induction of labor at term–a randomized controlled trial. *Wien Klin Wochenschr.* 113(23-24):942-6.
CONCLUSION(S): Acupuncture at points LI4 and SP 6 supports cervical ripening at term and can shorten the time interval between the EDC and the actual time of delivery.

Zeisler H, Tempfer C, Mayerhofer K, Barrada M, Husslein P. 1998. Influence of acupuncture on duration of labor. *Gynecol Obstet Invest.* 46(1):22-5.

CONCLUSION(S): This study suggests that AP treatment is a recommendable form of childbirth preparation due to its positive effect on the duration of labor, namely by shortening the first stage of labor.

7. Lactation and Acupuncture Research

Kvist LJ, Hall-Lord ML, Rydhstroem H, Larsson BW. 2007. A randomised-controlled trial in Sweden of acupuncture and care interventions for the relief of inflammatory symptoms of the breast during lactation. *Midwifery*. 23(2):184-95.
KEY CONCLUSIONS AND IMPLICATIONS FOR PRACTICE: If acupuncture treatment is acceptable to the mother, this, together with care interventions such as correction of breast feeding position and babies' attachment to the breast, might be a more expedient and less invasive choice of treatment than the use of oxytocin nasal spray. Midwives, nurses or medical practitioners with specialist competence in breast feeding should be the primary care providers for mothers with inflammatory symptoms of the breast during lactation. The use of antibiotics for inflammatory symptoms of the breast should be closely monitored in order to help the global community reduce resistance development among bacterial pathogens.

Neri I, Allais G, Vaccaro V, Minniti S, Airola G, Schiapparelli P, Benedetto C, Facchinetti F. 2011. Acupuncture treatment as breastfeeding support: preliminary data. *J Altern Complement Med*. 17(2):133-7.
CONCLUSION(S): Such preliminary data suggest that 3 weeks of acupuncture treatment were more effective than observation alone in maintaining breastfeeding until the third month of the newborns' lives.

Wei L, Wang H, Han Y, Li C. 2008. Clinical observation on the effects of electroacupuncture at Shaoze (SI 1) in 46 cases of postpartum insufficient lactation. *J Tradit Chin Med*. 28(3):168-72.
CONCLUSION(S): Electroacupuncture at Shaoze (SI 1) was obviously effective for postpartum insufficient lactation.

8. Male Factor Infertility Research

Dieterle S, Li C, Greb R, Bartzsch F, Hatzmann W, Huang D. 2009. A prospective randomized placebo-controlled study of the effect of acupuncture in infertile patients with severe oligoasthenozoospermia. *Fertil Steril*. 92(4):1340–3.
CONCLUSION(S): This recent small clinical trial randomized 57 patients who had extremely low sperm counts, to acupuncture and placebo acupuncture groups. After receiving acupuncture twice weekly for 6 weeks, motility of sperm (but not overall count) was found to increase significantly. The authors conclude that the results of the present study support the significance of acupuncture in male patients with severe oligoasthenozoospermia. More evidence with larger trials needs to be accumulated before the efficacy and effectiveness of acupuncture in male infertility can be evaluated.

Gurfinkel E, Cedenho AP, Yamamura Y, Srougi M. 2003. Effects of acupuncture
and moxa treatment in patients with semen abnormalities. *Asian J Androl.* 5(4):345-8.
CONCLUSION(S): The Chinese Traditional Medicine acupuncture and moxa techniques
significantly increase the percentage of normal-form sperm in patients with
oligoastenoteratozoospermia without apparent cause.

Pei J, Strehler E, Noss U, Abt M, Piomboni P, Baccetti B, Sterzik K. 2005.
Quantitative evaluation of spermatozoa ultrastructure after acupuncture treatment for
idiopathic male infertility. *Fertil Steril.* 84(1):141-7.
CONCLUSION(S): The treatment of idiopathic male infertility could benefit from
employing acupuncture. A general improvement of sperm quality, specifically in the
ultrastructural integrity of spermatozoa, was seen after acupuncture, although we did not
identify specific sperm pathologies that could be particularly sensitive to this therapy.

Siterman S, Eltes F, Schechter L, Maimon Y, Lederman H, Bartoov B. 2009.
Success of acupuncture treatment in patients with initially low sperm output is associated
with a decrease in scrotal skin temperature. *Asian J Androl.* 11(2):200-8.
CONCLUSION(S): Low sperm count in patients with inflammation of the genital tract
seems to be associated with scrotal hyperthermia, and, consequently, acupuncture
treatment is recommended for these men.

Siterman S, Eltes F, Wolfson V, Lederman H, Bartoov B. 2000. Does acupuncture
treatment affect sperm density in males with very low sperm count? A pilot study.
Andrologia. 32(1):31-9.
CONCLUSION(S): Acupuncture may be a useful, non-traumatic treatment for males
with very poor sperm density, especially those with a history of genital tract
inflammation.

Siterman S, Eltes F, Wolfson V, Zabludovsky N, Bartoov B. 1997. Effect of
acupuncture on sperm parameters of males suffering from subfertility related to low
sperm quality. *Arch Androl.* 39(2):155-61.
CONCLUSION(S): Patients exhibiting a low fertility potential due to reduced sperm
activity may benefit from acupuncture treatment.

9. PCOS and Acupuncture Research

Jedel E, Labrie F, Odén A, Holm G, Nilsson L, Janson PO, Lind AK, Ohlsson C,
Stener-Victorin E. 2011. Impact of electro-acupuncture and physical exercise on
hyperandrogenism and oligo/amenorrhea in women with polycystic ovary syndrome: a
randomized controlled trial. *Am J Physiol Endocrinol Metab.* 300(1):E37-45.
CONCLUSION(S): Low-frequency EA and physical exercise improved
hyperandrogenism and menstrual frequency more effectively than no intervention in
women with PCOS. Low-frequency EA was superior to physical exercise and may be
useful for treating hyperandrogenism and oligo/amenorrhea.

Johansson J, Redman L, Veldhuis PP, Sazonova A, Labrie F, Holm G, Johannsson

G, Stener-Victorin E. 2013. Acupuncture for ovulation induction in polycystic ovary syndrome: A randomized controlled trial. *Am J Physiol Endocrinol Metab.* 304(9): E934-43.
CONCLUSION(S): We conclude that repeated acupuncture treatments resulted in higher ovulation frequency in lean/overweight women with PCOS and were more effective than just meeting with the therapist. Ovarian and adrenal sex steroid serum levels were reduced with no effect on LH secretion.

Leonhardt H, Hellström M, Gull B, Lind AK, Nilsson L, Janson PO, Stener-Victorin E. 2015. Serum anti-Müllerian hormone and ovarian morphology assessed by magnetic resonance imaging in response to acupuncture and exercise in women with polycystic ovary syndrome: secondary analyses of a randomized controlled trial. *Acta Obstet Gynecol Scand.* 94(3):279-87.
CONCLUSION(S): This study is the first to demonstrate that acupuncture reduces serum AMH levels and ovarian volume. Physical exercise did not influence circulating AMH or ovarian volume. Despite a within-group decrease in AFC, exercise did not lead to a between-group difference.

Lim CE, Wong WS. 2010. Current evidence of acupuncture on polycystic ovarian syndrome. *Gynecol Endocrinol.* 26(6):473-8.
CONCLUSION(S): Acupuncture is a safe and effective treatment to PCOS as the adverse effects of pharmacologic interventions are not expected by women with PCOS. Acupuncture therapy may have a role in PCOS by: increasing of blood flow to the ovaries, reducing of ovarian volume and the number of ovarian cysts, controlling hyperglycaemia through increasing insulin sensitivity and decreasing blood glucose and insulin levels, reducing cortisol levels and assisting in weight loss and anorexia. However, well-designed, randomised controlled trials are needed to elucidate the true effect of acupuncture on PCOS.

Manneräs L, Jonsdottir IH, Holmäng A, Lönn M, Stener-Victorin E. 2008. Low-frequency electro-acupuncture and physical exercise improve metabolic disturbances and modulate gene expression in adipose tissue in rats with dihydrotestosterone-induced polycystic ovary syndrome. *Endocrinology.* 149(7):3559-68.
CONCLUSION(S): EA and exercise ameliorate insulin resistance in rats with PCOS. This effect may involve regulation of adipose tissue metabolism and production because EA and exercise each partly restore divergent adipose tissue gene expression associated with insulin resistance, obesity, and inflammation. In contrast to exercise, EA improves insulin sensitivity and modulates adipose tissue gene expression without influencing adipose tissue mass and cellularity.

Stener-Victorin E. 2013. Hypothetical physiological and molecular basis for the effect of acupuncture in the treatment of polycystic ovary syndrome. *Mol Cell Endocrinol.* 373(1-2):83-90.
ABSTRACT: Clinical and experimental evidence indicates that acupuncture may be a safe alternative or complement in the treatment of endocrine and reproductive function in women with polycystic ovary syndrome (PCOS). This review describes potential etiological factors of PCOS with the aim to support potential mechanism of action of acupuncture to relieve PCOS related symptoms. The theory that increased sympathetic

activity contributes to the development and maintenance of PCOS is presented, and that the effects of acupuncture are, at least in part, mediated by modulation of sympathetic outflow. While there are no relevant randomized controlled studies on the use of acupuncture to treat metabolic abnormalities in women with PCOS, a number of experimental studies indicate that acupuncture may improve metabolic dysfunction. For each aspect of PCOS, it is important to pursue new treatment strategies that have fewer negative side effects than drug treatments, as women with PCOS often require prolonged treatment.

10. Postpartum Depression and Acupuncture Research

Chung KF, Yeung WF, Zhang ZJ, Yung KP, Man SC, Lee CP, Lam SK, Leung TW, Leung KY, Ziea ET, Taam Wong V. 2012. Randomized non-invasive sham-controlled pilot trial of electroacupuncture for postpartum depression. *J Affect Disord.* 142(1-3):115-21. CONCLUSION(S): Both electroacupuncture and non-invasive sham acupuncture were effective for postpartum depression. Further studies utilizing larger sample size, better recruitment strategies, and home-based acupuncture treatment are warranted.

11. Pregnancy and Acupuncture Research

Ee CC, Manheimer E, Pirotta MV, White AR. 2008. Acupuncture for pelvic and back pain in pregnancy: a systematic review. *Am J Obstet Gynecol.* 198(3):254-9. ABSTRACT: The objective of our study was to review the effectiveness of needle acupuncture in treating the common and disabling problem of pelvic and back pain in pregnancy. Two small trials on mixed pelvic/back pain and 1 large high-quality trial on pelvic pain met the inclusion criteria. Acupuncture, as an adjunct to standard treatment, was superior to standard treatment alone and physiotherapy in relieving mixed pelvic/back pain. Women with well-defined pelvic pain had greater relief of pain with a combination of acupuncture and standard treatment, compared to standard treatment alone or stabilizing exercises and standard treatment. We used a narrative synthesis due to significant clinical heterogeneity between trials. Few and minor adverse events were reported. We conclude that limited evidence supports acupuncture use in treating pregnancy-related pelvic and back pain. Additional high-quality trials are needed to test the existing promising evidence for this relatively safe and popular complementary therapy.

Elden H, Ladfors L, Olsen MF, Ostgaard HC, Hagberg H. 2005. Effects of acupuncture and stabilising exercises as adjunct to standard treatment in pregnant women with pelvic girdle pain: randomised single blind controlled trial. *BMJ.* 330(7494):761. CONCLUSION(S): Acupuncture and stabilising exercises constitute efficient complements to standard treatment for the management of pelvic girdle pain during pregnancy. Acupuncture was superior to stabilising exercises in this study.

Manber R, Schnyer RN, Lyell D, Chambers AS, Caughey AB, Druzin M,

Carlyle E, Celio C, Gress JL, Huang MI, et al. 2010. Acupuncture for depression during pregnancy: a randomized controlled trial. *Obstet Gynecol.* 115(3):511-20.
CONCLUSION(S): The short acupuncture protocol demonstrated symptom reduction and a response rate comparable to those observed in standard depression treatments of similar length and could be a viable treatment option for depression during pregnancy.

Xu J, MacKenzie IZ. 2012. The current use of acupuncture during pregnancy and childbirth. *Curr Opin Obstet Gynecol.* 24(2):65-71.
CONCLUSION(S): Acupuncture therapy may offer some advantage over conventional treatment in the management of hyperemesis gravidarum and postcaesarean section pain and these areas warrant further study. Rigorous randomized studies, particularly those using objective measures, have failed to identify any obvious benefits from acupuncture for many of the other conditions studied.

Research Citations

Agarwal A, Desai NR, Makker K, Varghese A, Mouradi R, Sabanegh E, Sharma R. 2009. Effects of radiofrequency electromagnetic waves (RF-EMW) from cellular phones on human ejaculated semen: an in vitro pilot study. *Fertil Steril.* 92(4):1318-25.

Al-Kuran O, Al-Mehaisen L, Bawadi H, Beitawi S, Amarin Z. 2011. The effect of late pregnancy consumption of date fruit on labour and delivery. *J Obstet Gynaecol.* 31(1):29-31.

Al-Turki HA. 2015. Effect of smoking on reproductive hormones and semen parameters of infertile Saudi Arabians. *Urol Ann.* 7(1):63-6.

American Society of Nephrology. April 3, 2008. Evidence lacking on health benefits of drinking lots of water, according to review of literature. *ScienceDaily.*

Amin AF, Shaaban OM, Bediawy MA. 2008. N-acetyle cysteine for treatment of recurrent unexplained pregnancy loss. *Reprod Biomed Online.* 17(5):722-6.

Arlt W. 2004. Dehydroepiandrosterone and ageing. *Best Pract Res Clin Endocrinology.* 18(3):363-80.

[ASRM] Practice Committee of the American Society for Reproductive Medicine. 2012. Evaluation and treatment of recurrent pregnancy loss: a committee opinion. *Fertil Steril.* 98(5):1103–11.

Barad DH, Brill H, Gleicher N. 2007. Update on the use of dehydroepiandrosterone supplementation among women with diminished ovarian reserve. *J Assist Reprod Genet.* 24(12):629-34

Barad DH, Gleicher N. 2006. Effects of dehydroepiandrosterone on oocyte and embryo yields, embryo grade and cell number in IVF. *Hum Reprod.* 21(11):2845-9.

Barad DH, Gleicher N. 2005. Increased oocyte production after treatment with dehydroepiandrosterone. *Fertil Steril.* 84(756):1-3.

Ben-Meir A, Burstein E, Borrego-Alvarez A, Chong J, Wong E, Yavorska T, Naranian T, Chi M, Wang Y, Bentov Y, et al. 2015. Coenzyme Q10 restores oocyte mitochondrial function and fertility during reproductive aging. *Aging Cell.* 14(5):887-95. [Epub ahead of print]

Bentov Y, Casper RF. 2013. The aging oocyte – can mitochondrial function be improved? *Fertil Steril.* 99(1):18-22.

Bentov Y, Hannam T, Jurisicova A, Esfandiari N, Casper RF. 2014. Coenzyme Q10 supplementation and oocyte aneuploidy in women undergoing IVF-ICSI treatment. *Clin Med Insights Reprod Health.* 8(8):31-6.

Bhagavan, HN, Chopra RK. 2006. Coenzyme Q10: absorption, tissue uptake, metabolism and pharmacokinetics. *Free Radic Res.* 40(5):445-53.

Blencowe H, Cousens S, Modell B, Lawn J. 2010. Folic acid to reduce neonatal mortality from neural tube disorders. *Int J Epidemiol.* 39 Suppl 1:i110-21.

Blomberg Jensen, M. 2014. Vitamin D and male reproduction. *Nat Rev Endocrinol.* 10(3):175-86.

Bolúmar F, Olsen J, Rebagliato M, Bisanti L. 1997. Caffeine intake and delayed conception: a European multicenter study on infertility and subfecundity. *Am J Epidemiol.* 145(4):324-34.

Brand E. 2014. Pesticides and Chinese herbs: understanding the issues. *Acupuncture Today.* 15(6).

Buck Louis GM, Sundaram R, Sweeney AM, Schisterman EF, Maisog J, Kannan K. 2014. Urinary bisphenol A, phthalates, and couple fecundity: the Longitudinal Investigation of Fertility and the Environment (LIFE) Study. *Fertil Steril.* 101(5):1359-66.

Cabaton NJ, Wadia PR, Rubin BS, Zalko D, Schaeberle CM, Askenase MH, Gadbois JL, Tharp AP, Whitt GS, Sonnenschein C, Soto AM. 2011. Perinatal exposure to environmentally relevant levels of bisphenol A decreases fertility and fecundity in CD-1 mice. *Environ Health Perspect.* 119(4):547-52.

Cardini F, Weixin H. 1998. Moxibustion for correction of breech presentation: a randomized controlled trial. *JAMA.* 280(18):1580-4.

Casson PR, Lindsay MS, Pisarska MD, Carson SA, Buster JE. 2000. Dehydroepiandrosterone supplementation augments ovarian stimulation in poor responders: a case series. *Hum Reprod.* 15(10):2129-32.

Chavarro JE, Rich-Edwards JW, Rosner BA, Willett WC. 2008. Use of multivitamins, intake of B vitamins, and risk of ovulatory infertility. *Fertil Steril.* 49(4):289-93.

Chung KF, Yeung WF, Zhang ZJ, Yung KP, Man SC, Lee CP, Lam SK, Leung TW, Leung KY, Ziea ET, Taam Wong V. 2012. Randomized non-invasive sham-controlled pilot trial of electroacupuncture for postpartum depression. *J Affect Disord.* 142(1-3):115-21.

Citkovitz C, Klimenko E, Bolyai M, Applewhite L, Julliard K, Weiner Z. 2009. Effects of acupuncture during labor and delivery in a U.S. hospital setting: a case-control pilot study. *J Altern Complement Med.* 15(5):501-5.

Cohen S, Janicki-Deverts D, Doyle WJ, Miller GE, Frank E, Rabin BS, Turner RB. 2012. Chronic stress, glucocorticoid receptor resistance, inflammation, and disease risk. *PNAS.* 109(16):5995-9.

Czeizel AE, Dudas I. 1992. Prevention of the first occurrence of neural tube defects by periconceptional vitamin supplementation. *N Engl J Med.* 327(26):1832-5.

Dabrowski FA, Grzechocinska B, Wielgos M. 2015. The role of vitamin D in reproductive health—a Trojan Horse or the Golden Fleece? *Nutrients.* 7:4139-4153.

Dalman A, Eimani H, Sepehri H, Ashtiani SK, Valojerdi MR, Eftekhari-Yazdi P, Shahverdi A. 2008. Effect of mono-(2-ethylhexyl) phthalate (MEHP) on resumption of meiosis, in vitro maturation, and embryo development of immature mouse oocytes. *Biofactors.* 33(2):149-55.

Deghan Manshadi S, Ishiguro L, Sohn KJ, Medline A, Renlund R, Croxford R, Kim YI. 2014. Folic acid supplementation promotes mammary tumor progression in a rat model. *PLoS One*. 9(1):e84635.

Dudás I, Rockenbauer M, Czeizel AE. 1995. The effect of preconceptional multivitamin supplementation on the menstrual cycle. *Arch Gynecol Obstet*. 256(3):115-23.

Dumollard R, Carroll J, Duchen MR, Campbell K, Swann K. 2009. Mitochondrial function and redox state in mammalian embryos. *Semin Cell Dev Biol*. 20(3):346-53.

Esteves SC, Agarwal A. 2011. Novel concepts in male infertility. *Int Braz J Urol*. 37(1):5-15.

Fett, Rebecca. 2014. *It starts with the egg: how the science of egg quality can help you get pregnant naturally, prevent miscarriage, and improve your odds in IVF*. New York: Franklin Fox.

Firouzabadi RD, Rahmani E, Rahsepar M, Firouzabadi MM. 2014. Value of follicular fluid vitamin D in predicting pregnancy rate in an IVF program. *Arch Gynecol Obstet*. 289(1):201-6.

Fordney-Settlage D. 1981. A review of cervical mucus and sperm interactions in humans. *Int J Fertil*. 26(3):161-9.

Frosst P, Blom HJ, Milos R, Goyette P, Sheppard CA, Matthews RG, Boers GJ, den Heijer M, Kluijtmans LA, van den Heuvel LP, et al. 1995. A candidate genetic risk factor for vascular disease: a common mutation in methylenetetrahydrofolate reductase. *Nat Genet*. 10(1):111–113.

Fujimoto VY, Kim D, vom Saal FS, Lamb JD, Taylor JA, Bloom MS. 2011. Serum unconjugated bisphenol A concentrations in women may adversely influence oocyte quality during in vitro fertilization. *Fertil Steril*. 95(5):1816-9.

Galesanu C, Mocanu V. 2015. Vitamin D deficiency and the clinical consequences. *Rev Med Chir Soc Med Nat Iasi*. 119(2):310-8.

Gaskins AJ, Mumford SL, Chavarro JE, Zhang C, Pollack AZ, Wactawski-Wende J, Perkins NJ, Schisterman EF. 2012. The impact of dietary folate intake on reproductive function in premenopausal women: a prospective cohort study. *PLoS One*. 7(9):e46276.

Giammanco M, Di Majo D, La Guardia M, Aiello S, Crescimannno M, Flandina C, Tumminello FM, Leto G. 2015. Vitamin D in cancer chemoprevention. *Pharm Biol*. 53(10):1399-434.

Gleicher N, Barad DH. 2011. Dehydroepiandrosterone (DHEA) supplementation in diminished ovarian reserve (DOR). *Reprod Biol Endocrinol*. 17(9):67.

Gleicher N, Weghofer A, Barad DH. 2010. Dehydroepiandrosterone (DHEA) reduces embryo aneuploidy: direct evidence from preimplantation genetic screening (PGS). *Reprod Biol Endocrinol*. 10(8):140.

Greco E, Romano S, Iacobelli M, Ferrero S, Baroni E, Minasi MG, Ubaldi F, Rienzi L, Tesarik J. 2005. ICSI in cases of sperm DNA damage: beneficial effect of oral antioxidant treatment. *Hum Reprod*. 20(9):2590-4.

Gribel GP, Coca-Velarde LG, Moreira de Sá RA. 2011. Electro-acupuncture for cervical ripening prior to labor induction: a randomized clinical trial. *Arch Gynecol Obstet*. 283(6):1233-8.

Gudeloglu A, Parekattil S. 2013. Update in the evaluation of the azoospermic male. *Clinics*. 68(Suppl 1):27–34.

Gurzell EA, Teague H, Harris M, Clinthorne J, Shaikh SR, Fenton JI. 2013. DHA-enriched fish oil targets B cell lipid microdomains and enhances ex vivo and in vivo B cell function. *J Leukoc Biol*. 93(4):463-70.

Habek D, Cerkez Habek J, Jagust M. 2003. Acupuncture conversion of fetal breech presentation. *Fetal Diagn Ther.* 18(6):418-21.

Håkonsen LB, Ernst A, Ramlau-Hansen CH. 2014. Maternal cigarette smoking during pregnancy and reproductive health in children: a review of epidemiological studies. *Asian J Androl.* 16(1):39-49.

Harper AJ, Buster JE, Casson PR. 1999. Changes in adrenocorticol function with aging and therapeutic implications. *Semin Reprod Endocrinol.* 17(4):327-38.

Harper TC, Coeytaux RR, Chen W, Campbell K, Kaufman JS, Moise KJ, Thorp JM. 2006. A randomized controlled trial of acupuncture for initiation of labor in nulliparous women. *J Matern Fetal Neonatal Med.* 19(8):465-70.

Harris ES, Cao S, Littlefield BA, Craycroft JA, Scholten R, Kaptchuk T, Fu Y, Wang W, Liu Y, Chen H, et al. 2011. Heavy metal and pesticide content in commonly prescribed individual raw Chinese Herbal Medicines. *Sci Total Environ.* 409(20):4297-305.

Hullender Rubin LE, Opsahl MS, Wiemer KE, Mist SD, Caughey AB. 2015. Impact of whole systems traditional Chinese medicine on in vitro fertilization outcomes. *Reprod Biomed Online.* 30(6):602-12.

Hunt PA, Koehler KE, Susiarjo M, Hodges CA, Ilagan A, Voigt RC, Thomas S, Thomas BF, Hassold TJ. 2003. Bisphenol A exposure causes meiotic aneuploidy in the female mouse. *Curr Biol.* 13(7):546-53.

Hunt PA, Lawson C, Gieske M, Murdoch B, Smith H, Marre A, Hassold T, VandeVoort CA. 2012. Bisphenol A alters early oogenesis and follicle formation in the fetal ovary of the rhesus monkey. *PNAS.* 109(43):17525-30.

Ishizuka B, Kuribayashi Y, Murai K, Amemiya A, Itoh MT. 2000. The effect of melatonin on in vitro fertilization and embryo development in mice. *J Pineal Res.* 28(1):48-51.

Jacobs, PA, Hassold TJ. 1987. Chromosome abnormalities: origin and etiology in abortions and livebirths. In: Vogel F, Sperling K, editors. *Hum Gen.* Berlin: Springer-Verlag: 233–44.

Jahnke G, Marr M, Myers C, Wilson R, Travlos G, Price C. 1999. Maternal and developmental toxicity evaluation of melatonin administered orally to pregnant Sprague-Dawley rats. *Toxicol Sci.* 50(2):271-9.

Jung A, Schill WB, Schuppe HC. 2005. Improvement of semen quality by nocturnal scrotal cooling in oligozoospermic men with a history of testicular maldescent. *Int J Androl.* 28(2):93-8.

Kavanagh J, Kelly AJ, Thomas J. 2001. Sexual intercourse for cervical ripening and induction of labour. *Cochrane Database Syst Rev.* (2):CD003093.

Keller A, Litzelman K, Wisk LE, Maddox T, Cheng ER, Creswell PD, Witt WP. 2012. Does the perception that stress affects health matter? The association with health and mortality. *Health Psychol.* 31(5):677-84.

Kilic-Okman T, Kucuk M. 2004. N-acetyl-cysteine treatment for polycystic ovary syndrome. *Int J Gynaecol Obstet.* 85(3):296-7.

Kitamura S, Suzuki T, Sanoh S, Kohta R, Jinno N, Sugihara K, Yoshihara S, Fujimoto N, Watanabe H, Ohta S. 2005. Comparative study of the endocrine-disrupting activity of bisphenol A and 19 related compounds. *Toxicol Sci.* 84(2):249-59.

Klonoff-Cohen H, Bleha J, Lam-Kruglick P. 2002. A prospective study of the effects of female and male caffeine consumption on the reproductive endpoints of IVF and gamete intra-Fallopian transfer. *Hum Reprod.* 17(7):1746-54.

Knez J, Kranvogl R, Breznik BP, Vončina E, Vlaisavljević V. 2014. Are urinary bisphenol A levels in men related to semen quality and embryo development after medically assisted reproduction? *Fertil Steril.* 101(1):215-21.

Kulikauskas V, Blaustein D, Ablin RJ. 1985. Cigarette smoking and its possible effects on sperm. *Fertil Steril.* 44(4):526-8.

La Vignera S, Condorelli RA, Vicari E, D'Agata R, Calogero AE. 2012. Effects of the exposure to mobile phones on male reproduction: a review of the literature. *J Androl.* 33(3):350-6.

Lafuente R, González-Comadrán M, Solà I, López G, Brassesco M, Carreras R, Checa MA. 2013. Coenzyme Q10 and male infertility: a meta-analysis. *J Assist Reprod Genet.* 30(9):1147-56.

Lamb JD, Bloom MS, vom Saal FS, Taylor JA, Sandler JR, Fujimoto VY. 2008. Serum bisphenol A (BPA) and reproductive outcomes in couples undergoing IVF. *Fertil Steril.* 90:S186.

Lathi RB, Liebert CA, Brookfield KF, Taylor JA, vom Saal FS, Fujimoto VY, Baker VL. 2014. Conjugated bisphenol A in maternal serum in relation to miscarriage risk. *Fertil Steril.* 102(1):123-8.

Lazzarin N, Vaquero E, Exacoustos C, Bertonotti E, Romanini ME, Arduini D. 2009. Low-dose aspirin and omega-3 fatty acids improve uterine artery blood flow velocity in women with recurrent miscarriage due to impaired uterine perfusion. *Fertil Steril.* 92(1):296-300.

Lin LT, Tsui KH, Wang PH. 2015. Clinical application of dehydroepiandrosterone in reproduction: a review of the evidence. *J Chin Med Assoc.* 78(8):446-53.

Liu L, Trimarchi JR, Smith PJ, Keefe DL. 2002. Mitochondrial dysfunction leads to telomere attrition and genomic instability. *Aging Cell.* 1(1):40-6.

Louis GM, Lum KJ, Sundaram R, Chen Z, Kim S, Lynch CD, Schisterman EF, Pyper C. 2011. Stress reduces conception probabilities across the fertile window: evidence in support of relaxation. *Fertil Steril.* 95(7):2184-9.

Luck MR, Jeyaseelan I, Scholes RA. 1995. Ascorbic acid and fertility. *Biol Reprod.* 52(2):262-6.

Luk J, Torrealday S, Neal Perry G, Pal L. 2012. Relevance of vitamin D in reproduction. *Hum Reprod.* 27(10):3015-27.

Machtinger R, Orvieto R. 2014. Bisphenol A, oocyte maturation, implantation, and IVF outcome: review of animal and human data. *Reprod Biomed Online.* 29(4):404-10.

Magarelli PC, Cridennda DK, Cohen M. 2009. Changes in serum cortisol and prolactin associated with acupuncture during controlled ovarian hyperstimulation in women undergoing in vitro fertilization-embryo transfer treatment. *Fertil Steril.* 92(6):1870-9.

Mancini A, De Marinis L, Oradei A, Hallgass ME, Conte G, Pozza D, Littarru GP. 1994. Coenzyme Q10 concentrations in normal and pathological human seminal fluid. *J Androl.* 15(6):591-4.

Marquard K, Westphal LM, Milki AA, Lathi RB. 2010. Etiology of recurrent pregnancy loss in women over the age of 35 years. *Fertil Steril.* 94(4):1473-7.

Marra C, Pozzi I, Ceppi L, Sicuri M, Veneziano F, Regalia AL. 2011. Wrist-ankle acupuncture as perineal pain relief after mediolateral episiotomy: a pilot study. *J Altern Complement Med.* 17(3):239-41.

McNamara RK, Carlson SE. 2006. Role of omega-3 fatty acids in brain development and function: potential implications for the pathogenesis and prevention of psychopathology. *Prostaglandins Leukot Essent Fatty Acids.* 75(4-5):329-49.

Meeker JD, Hu H, Cantonwine DE, Lamadrid-Figueroa H, Calafat AM, Ettinger AS, Hernandez-Avila M, Loch-Caruso R, Téllez-Rojo MM. 2009. Urinary phthalate metabolites in relation to preterm birth in Mexico city. *Environ Health Perspect.* 117(10):1587-92.

Merhi ZO, Seifer DB, Weedon J, Adeyemi O, Holman S, Anastos K, Golub ET, Young M, Karim R, Greenblatt R, Minkoff H. 2012. Circulating vitamin D correlates with serum antimüllerian hormone levels in late-reproductive-aged women: Women's Interagency HIV Study. *Fertil Steril.* 98(1):228–34.

Momoi N, Tinney JP, Liu LJ, Elshershari H, Hoffmann PJ, Ralphe JC, Keller BB, Tobita K. 2008. Modest maternal caffeine exposure affects developing embryonic cardiovascular function and growth. *Am J Physiol Heart Circ Physiol.* 294(5): H2248-56.

Nabi H, Kivimäki M, Batty GD, Shipley MJ, Britton A, Brunner EJ, Vahtera J, Lemogne C, Elbaz A, Singh-Manoux A. 2013. Increased risk of coronary heart disease among individuals reporting adverse impact of stress on their health: the Whitehall II prospective cohort study. *Eur Heart J.* 34(34):2697-705.

Nasr A. 2010. Effect of N-acetyl-cysteine after ovarian drilling in clomiphene citrate-resistant PCOS women: a pilot study. *Reprod Biomed Online.* 20(3):403-9.

Nwhator SO, Opeodu OI, Ayanbadejo PO, Umeizudike KA, Olamijulo JA, Alade GO, Agbelusi GA, Arowojolu MO, Sorsa T. 2014. Could periodontitis affect time to conception? *Ann Med Health Sci Res.* 4(5):817–22.

O'Neill C. 1998. Endogenous folic acid is essential for normal development of preimplantation embryos. *Hum Reprod.* 13(5):1312–6.

Ozatik O, Aydin Y, Hassa H, Ulusoy D, Ogut S, Sahin F. 2013. Relationship between oxidative stress and clinical pregnancy in assisted reproductive technology treatment cycles. *J Assist Reprod Genet.* 30(6):765-72.

Ozkan S, Jindal S, Greenseid K, Shu J, Zeitlian G, Hickmon C, Pal L. 2010. Replete vitamin D stores predict reproductive success following in vitro fertilization. *Fertil Steril.* 94(4):1314-9.

Packer L, Witt EH, Tritschler HJ. 1995. Alpha-Lipoic acid as a biological antioxidant. *Free Radic Biol Med.* 19(2):227-50.

Paffoni A, Ferrari S, Viganò P, Pagliardini L, Papaleo E, Candiani M, Tirelli A, Fedele L, Somigliana E. 2014. Vitamin D deficiency and infertility: insights from in vitro fertilization cycles. *J Clin Endocrinol Metab.* 99(11):E2372-6.

Palioura E, Diamanti-Kandarakis E. 2013. Industrial endocrine disruptors and polycystic ovary syndrome. *J Endocrinol Invest.* 36(11):1105-11.

Pei J, Strehler E, Noss U, Abt M, Piomboni P, Baccetti B, Sterzik K. 2005. Quantitative evaluation of spermatozoa ultrastructure after acupuncture treatment for idiopathic male infertility. *Fertil Steril.* 84(1):141-7.

Poeggeler B, Reiter RJ, Tan DX, Chen LD, Manchester LC. 1993. Melatonin, hydroxyl radical-mediated oxidative damage, and aging, a hypothesis. *J Pineal Res.* 14(4):151-168.

Polak G, Koziol-Montewka M, Gogacz M, Błaszkowska I, Kotarski J. 2001. Total antioxidant status of peritoneal fluid in infertile women. *Eur J Obstet Gynecol Reprod Biol.* 94(2):261-3.

Polyzos NP, Anckaert E, Guzman L, Schiettecatte J, Van Landuyt L, Camus M, Smitz J, Tournaye H. 2014. Vitamin D deficiency and pregnancy rates in women undergoing single embryo, blastocyst stage, transfer (SET) for IVF/ICSI. *Hum Reprod.* 29(9):2032-40.

Richardson S, Shaffer JA, Falzon L, Krupka D, Davidson KW, Edmondson D. 2012. Meta-analysis of perceived stress and its association with incident coronary heart disease. *Am J Cardiol.* 110(12):1711-6.

Ried K, Stuart K. 2011. Efficacy of Traditional Chinese Herbal Medicine in the management of female infertility: a systematic review. *Complement Ther Med.* 19(6):319-31.

Ruder EH, Hartman TJ, Reindollar RH, Goldman MB. 2014. Female dietary antioxidant intake and time to pregnancy among couples treated for unexplained infertility. *Fertil Steril.* 101(3):759-66.

Rudick B, Ingles S, Chung K, Stanczyk F, Paulson R, Bendikson K. 2012. Characterizing the influence of vitamin D levels on IVF outcomes. *Hum Reprod.* 27(11):3321-7.

Rutkowska A, Rachoń D. 2014. Bisphenol A (BPA) and its potential role in the pathogenesis of the polycystic ovary syndrome (PCOS). *Gynecol Endocrinol.* 30(4):260-5.

Safarinejad MR. 2012. The effect of coenzyme Q10 supplementation on partner pregnancy rate in infertile men with idiopathic oligoasthenoteratozoospermia: an open-label prospective study. *Int Urol Nephrol.* 44(3):689-700.

Safarinejad MR, Hosseini SY, Dadkhah F, Asgari MA. 2010. Relationship of omega-3 and omega-6 fatty acids with semen characteristics, and antioxidant status of seminal plasma: a comparison between fertile and infertile men. *Clin Nutr.* 29(1):100-5.

Shigenaga MK, Hagen TM, Ames BN. 1994. Oxidative damage and mitochondrial decay in aging. *Proc Natl Acad Sci USA.* 91(23):10771-8.

Showell MG, Brown J, Clarke J, Hart RJ. 2013. Antioxidants for female subfertility. *Cochrane Database Syst Rev.* 8:CD007807.

Showell MG, Mackenzie-Proctor R, Brown J, Yazdani A, Stankiewicz MT, Hart RJ. 2014. Antioxidants for male subfertility. *Cochrane Database Syst Rev.* 12:CD007411.

Simerman AA, Hill DL, Grogan TR, Elashoff D, Clarke NJ, Goldstein EH, Manrriquez AN, Chazenbalk GD, Dumesic DA. 2015. Intrafollicular cortisol levels inversely correlate with cumulus cell lipid content as a possible energy source during oocyte meiotic resumption in women undergoing ovarian stimulation for in vitro fertilization. *Fertil Steril.* 103(1):249-57.

Stahlhut RW, Welshons WV, Swan SH. 2009. Bisphenol A data in NHANES suggest longer than expected half-life, substantial nonfood exposure, or both. *Environ Health Perspect.* 117(5):784-9.

Stojkovic M, Westesen K, Zakhartchenko V, Stojkovic P, Boxhammer K, Wolf E. 1999. Coenzyme Q(10) in submicron-sized dispersion improves development, hatching, cell proliferation, and adenosine triphosphate content of in vitro-produced bovine embryos. *Biol Reprod.* 61(2):541-7.

Swan SH, Main KM, Liu F, Stewart SL, Kruse RL, Calafat AM, Mao CS, Redmon JB, Ternand CL, Sullivan S, Teague JL; Study for Future Families Research Team. 2005. Decrease in anogenital distance among male infants with prenatal phthalate exposure. *Environ Health Perspect.* 113(8):1056-61.

Szymański W, Kazdepka-Ziemińska A. 2003. Effect of homocysteine concentration in follicular fluid on a degree of oocyte maturity. *Ginekol Pol.* 74(10):1392–6.

Takahashi O, Oishi S. 2000. Disposition of orally administered 2,2 Bis(4-hydroxyphenyl)propane (Bisphenol A) in pregnant rats and the placental transfer to fetuses. *Environ Health Perspect.* 108(10):931-5.

Tamura H, Takasaki A, Miwa I, Taniguchi K, Maekawa R, Asada H, Taketani T, Matsuoka A, Yamagata Y, Shimamura K, et al. 2008. Oxidative stress impairs oocyte quality and melatonin protects oocytes from free radical damage and improves fertilization rate. *J Pineal Res.* 44(3):280-7.

Tamura H, Takasaki A, Taketani T, Tanabe M, Kizuka F, Lee L, Tamura I, Maekawa R, Aasada H, Yamagata Y, Sugino N. 2012. The role of melatonin as an antioxidant in the follicle. *J Ovarian Res.* (5):5

Tatone C, Amicarelli F, Carbone MC, Monteleone P, Caserta D, Marci R, Artini PG, Piomboni P, Focarelli R. 2008. Cellular and molecular aspects of ovarian follicle ageing. *Hum Reprod Update.* 14(2):131-42.

Teh AL, Pan H, Chen L, Ong ML, Dogra S, Wong J, MacIsaac JL, Mah SM, McEwen LM, Saw SM, et al. 2014. The effect of genotype and in utero environment on interindividual variation in neonate DNA methylomes. *Genome Res.* 24(7):1064–74.

Tian YH, Baek JH, Lee SY, Jang CG. 2010. Prenatal and postnatal exposure to bisphenol A induces anxiolytic behaviors and cognitive deficits in mice. *Synapse.* 64(6):432-9.

Toft G, Jönsson BA, Lindh CH, Jensen TK, Hjollund NH, Vested A, Bonde JP. 2012. Association between pregnancy loss and urinary phthalate levels around the time of conception. *Environment Health Perspect.* 120(3):458-63.

Ueland PM, Hustad S, Schneede J, Refsum H, Vollset SE. 2001. Biological and clinical implications of the MTHFR C677T polymorphism. *Trends Pharmacol Sci.* 22(4):195–201.

Urman B, Yakin K. 2012. DHEA for poor responders: can treatment be justified in the absence of evidence? *Reprod Biomed Online.* 25(2):103-7.

Van Blerkom J, Davis PW, Lee J. 1995. ATP content of human oocytes and developmental potential and outcome after in-vitro fertilization and embryo transfer. *Hum Reprod.* 10(2):415-24.

Vandenberg LN, Chahoud I, Heindel JJ, Padmanabhan V, Paumgartten FJ, Schoenfelder G. 2012. Urinary, circulating, and tissue biomonitoring studies indicate widespread exposure to bisphenol A. *Cien Saude Colet.* 17(2):407-34.

van der Put NM, Steegers-Theunissen RP, Frosst P, Trijbels FJ, Eskes TK, van den Heuvel LP, Mariman EC, den Heyer M, Rozen R, Blom HJ. 1995. Mutated methylenetetrahydrofolate reductase as a risk factor for spina bifida. *Lancet.* 346(8982):1070–1.

Vas J, Aranda-Regules JM, Modesto M, Ramos-Monserrat M, Barón M, Aguilar I, Benítez-Parejo N, Ramírez-Carmona C, Rivas-Ruiz F. 2013. Using moxibustion in primary healthcare to correct non-vertex presentation: a multicentre randomised controlled trial. *Acupunct Med.* 31(1):31-8.

Vollset SE, Clarke R, Lewington S, Ebbing M, Halsey J, Lonn E, Armitage J, Manson JE, Hankey GJ, Spence JD, et al. 2013. Effects of folic acid supplementation on overall and site-specific cancer incidence during the randomised trials: meta-analyses of data on 50,000 individuals. *Lancet.* 381(9871):1029-36.

Wang W, Hafner KS, Flaws JA. 2014. In utero bisphenol A exposure disrupts germ cell nest breakdown and reduces fertility with age in the mouse. *Toxicol Appl Pharmacol.* 276(2):157-64.

Wdowiak A, Sulima M, Sadowska M, Grzegorz B, Bojar I. 2014. Alcohol consumption and quality of embryos obtained in programmes of in vitro fertilization. *Ann Agric Environ Med.* 21(2):450-3.

Wei L, Wang H, Han Y, Li C. 2008. Clinical observation on the effects of electroacupuncture at Shaoze (SI 1) in 46 cases of postpartum insufficient lactation. *J Tradit Chin Med.* 28(3):168-72.

Welshons WV, Nagel SC, vom Saal FS. 2006. Large effects from mall exposures. III. Endocrine mechanisms mediating effects of bisphenol A at levels of human exposure. *Endocrinology.* 147(6 Suppl):S56-69.

Weng X, Odouli R, Li DK. 2008. Maternal caffeine consumption during pregnancy and the risk of miscarriage: a prospective cohort study. *Am J Obstet Gynecol.* 198(3):279.e1-8.

Wilding M, Dale B, Marino M, di Matteo L, Alviggi C, Pisaturo ML, Lombardi L, De Placido G. 2001. Mitochondrial aggregation patterns and activity in human oocytes and preimplantation embryos. *Hum Reprod.* 16(5):909-17.

Wilding M, De Placido G, De Matteo L, Marino M, Alviggi C, Dale B. 2003. Chaotic mosaicism in human preimplantation embryos is correlated with a low mitochondrial membrane potential. *Fertil Steril.* 79(2):340-6.

Wong WY, Merkus HM, Thomas CM, Menkveld R, Zielhuis GA, Steegers-Theunissen RP. 2002. Effects of folic acid and zinc sulfate on male factor subfertility: a double-blind, randomized, placebo-controlled trial. *Fertil Steril.* 77(3):491-8.

[WHO] World Health Organization. 2009. *Pesticide residues in food - 2007, toxicological evaluations: joint FAO/WHO meeting on pesticide residues.* Geneva (Switzerland): WHO Press.

Yakin K, Urman B. 2011. DHEA as a miracle drug in the treatment of poor responders: hype or hope? *Hum Reprod.* 26(8):1941-4.

Zeisler H, Tempfer C, Mayerhofer K, Barrada M, Husslein P. 1998. Influence of acupuncture on duration of labor. *Gynecol Obstet Invest.* 46(1):22-5.

Zembron-Lacny A, Slowinska-Lisowska M, Szygula Z, Witkowski K, Szyszka K. 2009. The comparison of antioxidant and hematological properties of N-acetylcysteine and alpha-lipoic acid in physically active males. *Physiol Res.* 58(6):855-861.

Zhang X, Wu XQ, Lu S, Guo YL, Ma X. 2006. Deficit of mitochondria-derived ATP during oxidative stress impairs mouse MII oocyte spindles. *Cell Res.* 16(10):841-50.

Photo Credits

Most of the photos in this book, excluding the cover illustrations, photos of the authors, and logos, are from www.dreamstime.com. Cover illustrations by Juli Douglas. Author photos by Jason McRuer.

About The Authors

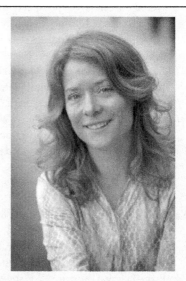

Stephanie Gianarelli, LAc, FABORM

As a fertility acupuncturist, it is my honor to assist women and their partners in their pursuit to become parents. I see parenthood as a sacred journey, and it's my job to help them prepare for that journey by assisting them in becoming as healthy as possible in body, mind, and spirit. Not only does getting healthier often increase your chances of becoming pregnant, but according to the tenets of Chinese medicine, healthier parents make healthier children. And that's my goal.

Stephanie Gianarelli (LAc, Dipl.Ac, Dipl.CH) is a Fellow of the American Board of Oriental Reproductive Medicine (ABORM) and a licensed and national board certified acupuncturist and Chinese herbalist. Stephanie received her Master's degree in Oriental Medicine from Southwest Acupuncture College in Santa Fe, New Mexico in 1999. She also completed postgraduate training in acupuncture and Chinese herbology focusing on gynecology at Zhe Jiang University of Traditional Chinese Medicine in Hang Zhou, P.R. China. She founded Acupuncture Northwest in Seattle, Washington in 2000, in the same building it is still in today.

Acupuncture Northwest & Associates is the Northwest's premier fertility enhancement acupuncture clinic. Stephanie Gianarelli and Acupuncture Northwest & Associates have been featured in the *Seattle Times*, KING 5's *Evening Magazine*, KOMO 4 News, *Alternative Medicine Magazine, South Sound Magazine,* and *Seattle Magazine*. Acupuncture Northwest and Associates' expert practitioners have also written articles for *RESOLVE's* national publication and *Family Building Magazine,* and they have given presentations across the Puget Sound region for groups as prestigious as the Seattle OB/GYN Society and for *RESOLVE's* annual Northwest conference.

Acupuncture Northwest & Associates has, by far, the highest concentration of nationally certified fertility acupuncturists in Washington State. The clinics have specialized in fertility enhancement and pregnancy for more than 10 years, and its acupuncturists are nationally board certified fertility acupuncturists with the American Board of Oriental Reproductive Medicine (ABORM). In addition, acupuncturists at Acupuncture Northwest & Associates work closely with local reproductive endocrinologists (fertility doctors), OB/GYNs, and midwives.

Acupuncture Northwest & Associates is a member of RESOLVE, the American Board of Oriental Reproductive Medicine (ABORM), and the American Society of Reproductive Medicine (ASRM).

For more information about Acupuncture Northwest and its individual practitioners, please visit our website at acupuncturenorthwest.com.

Lora Shahine, MD, FACOG

As a reproductive endocrinologist, I provide the kind of care I would want for myself, my family, and friends. Difficulty having a family is an intimate and personal challenge—medically and emotionally. I provide a caring, personal approach in a practice which provides the most advanced technology, up to date care, and high success rates.

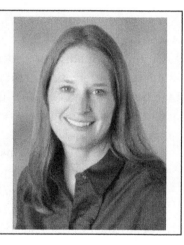

Lora Shahine, MD, FACOG, practices at Pacific NW Fertility and IVF Specialists in Seattle, WA, and completed her fellowship in Reproductive Endocrinology and Infertility at Stanford University. During her time at Stanford, Dr. Shahine served as a Clinical Instructor in the department of Obstetrics and Gynecology, contributed to several research publications on women's health and infertility, and trained in one of the few Centers for Recurrent Pregnancy Loss in the United States.

Dr. Shahine is board certified in Reproductive Endocrinology and Infertility as well as in Obstetrics and Gynecology. She is a fellow in The American College of Obstetrics and Gynecology and a member of The American Society of Reproductive Medicine (ASRM), The Washington State Obstetrical Association, The Seattle Gynecology Society, and The Pacific Coast Reproductive Society.

Dr. Shahine earned her MD at Wake Forest University School of Medicine in North Carolina, where she received the Faculty Award for outstanding academic and clinical achievement and was inducted in the national medical school honor society, Alpha Omega Alpha.

She completed her residency in Obstetrics and Gynecology at the University of California at San Francisco (UCSF) where she was honored with teaching awards for her dedication to mentoring medical students and other residents and received the Jim Green Award for outstanding clinical and research achievement in residency upon graduation.

As the Director of the Pacific NW Fertility Recurrent Pregnancy Loss Program, Dr. Shahine provides up to date, thorough, and personalized care for individuals suffering from multiple miscarriages. Dr. Shahine feels that the inability to carry a pregnancy to term is a unique type of infertility, and she is dedicated to helping patients every step of the way as they build their family.

- ❏ Board Certified in Obstetrics & Gynecology
- ❏ Board Certified in Reproductive Endocrinology and Infertility
- ❏ Subspecialty training/fellowship in Reproductive Endocrinology & Infertility – Stanford University
- ❏ Residency in Obstetrics and Gynecology at the University of California at San Francisco
- ❏ Doctor of Medicine from Wake Forest University School of Medicine, Winston-Salem, NC
- ❏ Member of the Pacific Coast Reproductive Society and the American Society of Reproductive Medicine
- ❏ Fellow of the American College of Obstetrics and Gynecology
- ❏ Clinical Faculty in the Department of Obstetrics and Gynecology at University of Washington

Acknowledgements

We want to thank Juli Douglas of Juli Douglas Illustration for her fine cover illustrations. You can reach her at www.julidouglas.com.

We would also like to thank Lucy Elenbaas for her wonderful editing skills. She really brought this book together. You can reach her at lucycarolineelenbaas.wordpress.com.

And thank you to the amazing writer and editor Cathy Beyer, who taught Stephanie one writing class in college and has read everything she has written since.

Index

Acupuncture	**13**, 14, 25, 26, 65-67, 113
-Postpartum	**93-94**, 126
-Research	118-132, 134, 135
-With ART	83, **84-85**, 120-122
-With Pregnancy	**87-93**, 126-127
Adenosine Triphosphate (ATP)	44, 53, **113**, 134, 135
Alcohol	23, **28**, 32, 34, 62, 94, 101, 134
Alpha Lipoic Acid	47, **48-49**, 113, 132, 135
American Board of Obstetricians and Gynecologists (ACOG)	**111**
American Board of Oriental Reproductive Medicine (ABORM)	**110**
Aneuploid	44, **113**, 128, 129, 130
Anti-Inflammatory Foods	**29-30**
Anti-Müllerian Hormone (AMH)	8, 42-43, 70, **71**, 111, 114, 115, 125
Antioxidants	29-30, **47-49**, 54, 113, 129, 132-135
Antral Follicle Count	70, **71**, 73, 113, 114
Assisted Reproductive Technology (ART)	29, 36, **69-82**, 113, 121, 131-132
-And TCM	15, 35, **83-86**
-Procedures	**72-82**
-Testing	**69-72**
Baby Bank Account	**21-23**, 28
Basal Body Temperature (BBT)	8, 57, **60-64**, 113
Blastocyst	44, 50, **113**, 120, 132
Blood Deficiency	65, **99-100**
Blood Sugar	**27-28**, 49, 87, 89
Bone Broth	**28**
BPA	32, **50-52**, 54, 131, 133
Breech	6, **90-91**, 118-119, 128, 130
Caffeine	22, 23, **29**, 94, 128, 130, 132, 135
Cervical Factor Infertility	75, 114
Cervical Fluid (Mucus)	13, **58-59**, 62, 129
Chinese Herbal Medicine	8, 11, 16, **34-35**, 67, 89
-And Pesticides	**108-109**, 128
-Research	**119**, 120, 121, 130, 133
-With ART	35, **85-86**
Chromosomes	**37-38**, 44, 82, 113

Clomid	73-74
Coenzyme Q10	**44-45**, 127, 128, 131, 133
Coffee	**29**, 32, 52
Cruciferous Vegetables	**30**
Cryopreservation	**79-80**, 114, 117
Cysts	15, 70, 74, 116, 125
Deficiency	
-Blood	65, **99-100**
-Jing/Essence	16, **22**, 29
-Yang	63, **97-98**
-Yin	**96-97**
DHEA	**45-47**, 129, 134, 135
Digestion	13, 20, 104-105, **106-107**
Diminished Ovarian Reserve (DOR)	8, 15, **36-8**, 43, 45-46, 71, 79, 114, 127, 129
Donor Egg	8, 36, **79**
Egg Quality	6, 9, **36-38**, 55, 129
-And ART	70, 78-79
-And Toxins	51
-With Supplements	38, 40, 43-47, 49, 50
-With TCM	15, **21-22**
Essence (Jing)	16, **20-24**, 28, 29, 114
Exercise	
-Postpartum	95
-Pre-Conception	23, 30, **33-34**
-Research	124, 125, 126
-Second Trimester	89
-With Self-Diagnosis	98, 100
Fats	27, 28
FDA	39-40, 74
Femara (Letrozole)	73-74
Fibroids	70
Folate	31, **40-42**, 129, 134
Folic Acid	**40-42**, 128, 129, 132, 134, 135
Follicle-Stimulating Hormone (FSH)	**71**, 73, 74, 77, 114, 115
Follicular Phase	61, 73, 113, **114**, 116
Follistim	74
Four Pillars of TCM Treatment	**25**, 114, 117
Genetic Screening/Testing	72, **81-82**, 129
Gonadotropins	37, **74**, 77, 115
Gonal-F	74
Green Tea	29, 30

Heart Organ System	20
History of TCM	11-12
Hysterosalpingogram (HSG)	66, **70**, 115
Intracytoplasmic Sperm Injection (ICSI)	77-78, 115
Intrauterine Insemination (IUI)	6, 12, 33, 69, 72-73, **74-76**, 85, 113, 115
In Vitro Fertilization (IVF)	15, 36, 72, **76-79**, 84-85, 113, 115, 121, 129-134
Jing (see Essence)	
Kidney Organ System	**20-24**
Labor Preparation	**90-93**, 122-123
Lactation	93, 94, 123, 134
Liver Organ System	18, **19**
Lung Organ System	20
Luteal Phase	57, 61, 63, 73, 76, 115
Luteal Phase Defect	15, 115
Luteinizing Hormone (LH)	59, 75, 115, 116
Male Factor	36, **53-55**, 77, 78
-ART	77, 78
-Research	123-124, 128, 129, 135
-Supplements	43, 54-55
Marijuana	34
Melatonin	47, **49-50**, 113, 130, 132, 134
Menstrual Cycle	13, 15, 36, 56, **57**, 60, 72, 73, 119, 120, 129
Meridians	13, 66, 67, 115, 116
Middle Burner	**106-107**
Miscarriage	8, 138
-Egg Quality	37-38
-Nutrition	29
-Research	129, 131, 135
-Supplements	49
-TCM	87-89
-Toxins	32, 51, 52
-Western Screening	72, 82
Morning Sickness	**88**, 89
Moxibustion	6, 26, 88, 91, **115**, 118, 119, 120, 128, 134
MTHFR	**41**, 134
Multivitamin	30-31, 40, 54, 129
N-Acetylcysteine (NAC)	47, **49**, 113, 135
Natural Conception	9, 42, **56-64**, 73
Nicotine	**33**, 94
Nutrition	**27-32**, 83, 84, 94, 96-103, 104-105

Omega-3 Fatty Acids	30, 31, 131, 133
Oral Hygiene	**33**
Organ Systems	**17-24**
-Heart	**20**
-Kidneys	**20-24**
-Liver	18, **19**
-Lung	**20**
-Spleen	18, **20**
Organic Foods	27, 28, 32, 42
Ovarian Hyperstimulation Syndrome (OHSS)	80, 116, 121
Ovarian Reserve	**36-37**, 43, 113, 114, **116**
-ART	79
-Research	127, 129
-Supplements	38, 43, 45-46
-TCM	15
-Testing	70-72
Ovulation	15, 37, 40, 44, 49, 50, **57-61**, 63-64, 116
-Research	119, 120, 125
-TCM	19, 26,
-TCM & ART	85
-Western Treatment	**72-76**, 77
Ovulation Predictor Kits (OPKs)	57, **59**, 60, 75, 76, 116
PCOS	12, 15, 49, 51, 116, 121, 124-126, 132, 133
Peak Day	**58-59**
Phthalates	32, 50, 51, **52-53**, 54, 128
Postpartum	12, **93-95**, 123, 126, 128, 134
Postpartum Depression	93, 94, 126, 128
Pregnancy	12, 19, 29, 42, 51-52, 64, 126-127, 130, 133, 135
-1st Trimester	80, **87-89**
-2nd Trimester	**89-90**
-3rd Trimester	**90-92**
-Labor	**90-93**, 122-123, 128, 129, 130, 135
Preimplantation Genetic Diagnosis	**81-82**, 116
Premature Ovarian Failure (POF)	15, 79, 116
Premenstrual Symptoms (PMS)	13, 19, 62
Prolactin	22, 72, 121, 131
Qi	**13**, 18, 20, 21-23, 66, 94, 114, 115, **116**
Recurrent Pregnancy Loss (RPL)	15, 117, 127, 131, 137-138

Research (Acupuncture and
     Chinese Herbal Medicine)   118-135▯
     -Blood Flow   118
     -Breech   118-119
     -Chinese Herbal Medicine   119
     -Female Fertility   120
     -IVF   120-122
     -Labor Preparation   122-123
     -Lactation   123
     -Male Factor   123-124
     -PCOS   124-126
     -Postpartum Depression   126
     -Pregnancy   126-127
Rubella Titers   72
Semen Analysis   16, 55, 70, **71**
Sleep   13, 22, **32, 33, 34**, 45, 48, 65, 99, 105
     -With an Infant   94
     -With a TCM Diagnosis   97, 99, 100, 101
     -With BBT   61
     -With Pregnancy   89, 90, 93
Sperm   9, **53-55**, 117
     -And Acupuncture   26, 37-38, 84-85
     -And Chinese Medicine   12, 16, 21, 83-86
     -And Labor   93
     -And Lifestyle   34
     -And Natural Conception   56-60
     -And Nutrition   27
     -And Smoking   33
     -And Supplements   31, 44
     -And Toxins   51
     -And Western Treatment   71-80, 115
     -Research   123-124, 129, 130, 131, 132, 133
     -Testing   71
Spleen Organ System   18, **20**
Stress   4, 5, 30, **32-33**, 34, 58, 62
     -And Pregnancy   89-90, 93
     -And TCM   13, 15, 16, 18, 19, 23, 100, 101
     -Oxidative   44, 47, 49-50, 54, 113, 132, 135
     -Research   128, 130, 131, 132, 133
Supplements   8, 25, 27, **38-50**, 53, 67, 84, 92
     -Alpha Lipoic Acid   47, **48-49**, 113, 132, 135

-Coenzyme Q10	**44-45**, 127, 128, 131, 133
-DHEA	**45-47**, 129, 134, 135
-Fish Oil	27, **30-31**, 54, 129
-Melatonin	47, **49-50**, 113, 130, 132, 134
-N-Acetylcysteine (NAC)	47, **49**, 113, 135
Thyroid	30, 49, 72, 99
Toxins	4, 18, 19, 32, 34, 38, 50-53, 54, 108
Traditional Chinese Medicine (TCM)	
-Diagnoses	
-Blood Deficiency	65, **99-100**
-Dampness	66, **103**
-Essence/Jing Deficiency	16, 22
-Excess Heat	65, **102**
-Heart Deficiency	**101-102**
-Kidney Yang Deficiency	63, **97-98**
-Kidney Yin Deficiency	**96-97**
-Liver Qi Stagnation	19, **100-101**
-Spleen Qi Deficiency	**98-99**
-With ART	15, 35, **83-86**, 120-122
-IUI	84-86
-IVF	84-86
Trigger Shot (HCG)	**75-76**
Ultrasound	66, 70, 75, 76, 77, 113, 117
-Pelvic	70
-Transvaginal	75, 77, 113, 117
Uterine Blood Flow	118, 121, 131
Varicella Titers	72
Varicocele	16, 54, 117
Vitamins	
-Folate	31, **40-42**, 129, 134
-Folic Acid	**40-42**, 128, 129, 132, 134, 135
-Multivitamin	30-31, 39-40, 54, 129
-Prenatal Vitamin	31
-Vitamin C	40, 47, **48-49**, 54, 113
-Vitamin D	27, **42-43**, 128, 129, 131, 132, 133
-Vitamin E	47, **48**, 54, 113
-Zinc	30, **54**, 135
Vitrification	**79-80**, 117
Zinc	30, **54**, 135

Made in the USA
Monee, IL
23 August 2020